A
Life
in
Medicine

For Tona, to whom I owe so much

EOIN O'BRIEN

A
Life
in
Medicine

From

ASCLEPIUS

to

BECKETT

THE LILLIPUT PRESS
DUBLIN

First published 2023 by
THE LILLIPUT PRESS

62–63 Sitric Road, Arbour Hill
Dublin 7, Ireland
www.lilliputpress.ie

ISBN 978 184351 8686

10 9 8 7 6 5 4 3 2 1

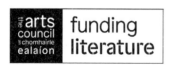

The Lilliput Press gratefully acknowledges the financial support of the Arts Council/ An Chomhairle Ealaíon.

Set in 11pt on 15pt Garamond with Frutiger display by Compuscript
Printed in Kerry by Walsh Colour Print

Contents

Illustrations between pages 116 and 117.

Author's Note

Once there is speech, no need of a story, a story is not compulsory, just a life, that's the mistake I made, one of the mistakes, to have wanted a story for myself, whereas life alone is enough.
Samuel Beckett, *Stories and Texts for Nothing* (1946)

To claim my past, scour it and do with it as I wish seemed at first to be my inalienable right. But when I began to put my past together, I realized I owned little of it. It was as if my history existed courtesy of others, and I was merely a spectator. The peregrinations of life happened not always at my behest but rather under the aegis of the teachers who dominated my formative years in school and medicine, and the scientists, artists and writers I later befriended.

Although many famous people drift across these pages, obscure figures, who would never find mention in the annals of history, but whose presence was influential in my life, do so too. Likewise, the institutional influences of schooling and medical training that may have escaped historical attention are given consideration.

Having been a physician for over half a century, I have witnessed remarkable advances in medical science: diseases such as rheumatic fever and tuberculosis that were often fatal when I began to study, are no longer prevalent in affluent countries. Surgical procedures such as coronary artery stenting and keyhole surgery are now commonplace. Yet the evolution of these dramatic advances, as they occurred on the ward or in the emergency departments of hospitals, has not often been given expression simply because doctors and nurses are busy people whose writing is confined to hospital notes or scientific journals, with the mundane, yet revelatory, happenings of day-to-day existence passing unnoticed.

In this memoir I focus on my life as a doctor in active clinical practice and I have not given consideration to the endeavours I became associated with in my retirement.

Doctors need to escape from medicine! Some of my colleagues became golfers or sailors, others became opera or theatre followers, and some became writers. I was drawn to the beauty of artistic expression, be it in literature, painting or music. This fascination brought me into the company of wonderful people who welcomed me to a world removed from the practice of medicine but which, nonetheless, often enhanced my understanding of human frailty and illness. These friends, who took me away from the wards, occupy a special place in this exploration of past times.

– Eoin O'Brien, Sandycove, County Dublin, January 2023

Foreword by John Banville

In this splendid memoir Eoin O'Brien recuperates a vanished world, if only in words. But what is 'only' about words? They are where we live, and where the past endures. Memory is notoriously undependable in the matter of places and events, but what has been written, as the poet Horace assured us, will outlast the Pyramids.

When he came to contemplate and organize his own past, Professor O'Brien observes with some surprise how little of it he owns – 'It was as if my history existed courtesy of others, and I was merely a spectator.' One understands the sentiment, but begs to differ. The record here of a life and the times in which it was lived is a rich and varied tapestry, and the weaver of it was, and is, for all his doubts, a highly active participant.

His narrative opens with a delightful recollection of sitting as a little boy on the knee of his paternal grandfather – 'old man with stick', as he was known to his grandchildren – in a prelapsarian, sunlit garden on the North Circular Road. It is an image emblematic of the life the little boy would go on to live, which from his account of it has known more brightness than shadow. 'If I were to define life as a gamble, it is fair to say I was dealt a pretty good hand.'

The opening chapters, dealing with his family origins and his childhood, provide a fascinating account of the aspirations and achievements of determined people in a poverty-stricken and often repressive nascent state – younger readers will hardly credit the struggles that were required by intelligent and public-spirited individuals to make a living, and a life, in the first half of the twentieth century, before and especially after the foundation of the Republic.

'I grew up,' Professor O'Brien tells us, 'in proximity to nurses, doctors and patients.' Both his parents were physicians. They were bright, diligent and hard-working, but both encountered disappointment and even betrayal in their careers. His father's early contribution to the battle against tuberculosis, the scourge of the times, went largely unacknowledged, leaving him emotionally astray in his later years. All the same, Professor O'Brien tells us, 'GT', as his father was known, 'dominates my reminiscences'.

The professor's mother, Muriel, or 'Moo', which was the family's affectionate nickname for her, studied at the Royal College of Surgeons in Ireland, securing top marks in her examinations, and in 1934 was presented with a gold medal as leading House Physician at Mercer's Hospital in Dublin. She gave up medicine after a young patient whom she was attending died accidentally, and legal action was taken, the result of which is unknown to the author. 'She never spoke of this incident,' he writes, 'which I uncovered in her papers after her death.' What family has not its secret sorrows?

The young Eoin O'Brien had a knack for getting into trouble. And in those authoritarian times, trouble was easy to get into. One day for a prank he and a couple of friends went into an Anglican church on Clyde Road and paraded, chanting, down the aisle. They were surprised by the vicar, who marched them to their Catholic-run school and denounced them to the headmaster, who had no choice but to expel the trio. Why so severe a punishment? Because the Archbishop of Dublin, the poisonous and all-powerful John Charles McQuaid, had forbidden Catholics to enter a Protestant Church under pain of excommunication. Ah, yes, Dublin in the rare oul times…

Life in the city in the 1950s was at once pinched and colourful. Doctors, nurses and medical students were something of a special breed, acknowledged as dedicated professionals at work, but envied as unsubduably racy once outside the hospital, the surgery or the college. Medicine at that time was still a 'hands-on' practice, actually as well as figuratively. Professor O'Brien shows us a closed world that is closer to the Holles Street Hospital episode in *Ulysses* than to the present-day, largely impersonal and mechanized business of treating the sick. These pages abound in medical 'characters', physicians who were as eccentric as they were caring.

But not as eccentric as the denizens of Baggotonia, that fabled area of the city that 'stretched from the Grand Canal towards the city along Baggot Street with its meagre flats and studios, past the parks of Fitzwilliam and Merrion to St Stephen's Green and onwards to Grafton Street.' It was here that literary Dublin based itself. Eoin O'Brien specialized in cardiology, but his love was for writing and writers and painting and painters.

One of the odd things about Baggotonia – and there were many – is the fact that most of the writers who haunted it were not Dubliners, but 'up from the Country'. Brendan Behan was the chief exception. Others, such as Patrick Kavanagh, Flann O'Brien, Ben Kiely, John McGahern – who would have objected to being considered a Baggotonian, though he spent much time there – and many more, had shaken the rural dust from their heels and fled to the city. The result was that the indigenous Irish literature of the time – that is, produced by those who had not emigrated, or 'gone into exile', as they would have insisted, such as Joyce and Beckett – had a strong pastoral flavour, even when its setting was urban.

It is to Beckett that Professor O'Brien's final chapter is devoted. They were friends from 1977, when the two first met, until 1989, the year of the writer's death. These pages are suffused with a fondness and warmth that emanated from both sides of the friendship. Readers who make the mistake of seeing the whole man through the dark glass of his work may be surprised by this portrait of a supposedly unrelenting pessimist, but they should not be. The Beckett we encounter here is a great artist, and a kindly, affable and mischievously humorous human being.

This is a fascinating, affecting and oddly bracing memoir. It celebrates, and commemorates, both the things of the mind and of the world. In places it is angry – this physician did not always see eye to eye with the Irish medical establishment – and in places wistful, but in all its parts it is grandly affirmative. We began by invoking Horace, and we shall make an end by suggesting that a fitting epigraph for the book might be provided by the Roman poet: 'Tomorrow do thy worst, for I have lived today.'

I

1. *Family Origins*

We are survival machines – robot vehicles blindly programmed to preserve
the selfish molecules known as genes. This is a truth which still fills me with
astonishment.
Richard Dawkins, *The Selfish Gene* (1976)

We are all moulded by our genes, those little pieces of magical transference. Our
genetic composition, modified over time by environmental influences, determines,
to a large extent, our destiny. I don't need Mendel, or Crick and Watson, to prove
the science of genetic expression to me – I need only observe myself; looking in
the mirror year by year, I begin to resemble the man who was my father.

The subtlety of genetic penetrance is fascinating. My handwriting, for
example, never resembled my father's until I passed the age of sixty; then his and
my signatures became almost indistinguishable. So, a dollop of DNA had lain
dormant for over half a century awaiting its moment of expression, and suddenly
there it was – manifest in a signature! Without becoming embroiled in a genetic
exegesis, I've been driven, nonetheless, to delve into the past of my parents and
their parents to discern the influences, both genetic and behavioural, that may
have contributed to my formation.

In my youth, I believed I hailed from the small town of Ennistymon in County Clare: this topographical error arose from the mistaken belief that my paternal grandfather was a Clare man, whereas he had merely served in that county as a member of the Royal Irish Constabulary (RIC) – the first force to provide policing in Ireland from the early nineteenth century until 1922.[1] The truth is that my paternal origins rest in the little town of Clonmellon in County Westmeath, where the O'Briens had been resident from at least the mid-nineteenth century, and where my paternal grandfather was born in 1857.[2] That my great-grandparents made use of the emerging medium of photography to portray a handsome couple is testimony to a modest degree of affluence and eminence.

I have only one warm memory of my paternal grandfather, a kindly man, known by his grandchildren as 'old man with stick', who sat me on his knee one summer's day, in the garden of his daughter's house on the North Circular Road in Dublin. The sun shone from a cloudless sky which warmed us in the shade of an apple tree. He had picked the ripest strawberries and removed the stalk and all vestiges of greenery before allowing me to guzzle the fruit. I can still smell the strawberries – none since have ever tasted so good – and the aroma of pipe tobacco from the striped flannel shirt that offered a resting place for my head and an embracing safeness. Then, he would be dead within a year, in his ninetieth year, when I was in my seventh, but his warmth and enduring presence impelled me to learn more about this remarkable man, who not only lived in a different time but who also occupied a land so changed by circumstance that it would now be unrecognizable to him.

Like so many of his generation, my grandfather's overriding ambition was to secure education for his children so that they might overcome the obstacles of poverty and ignorance inflicted on the country over centuries of British rule. The sacrifices that parents of this era made to ensure that their offspring were educated are astounding and account in large measure for the success of modern Ireland. Was it proximity to the Penal Laws and the hedge schools, the cessation of Protestant proselytizing with the advent of Catholic Emancipation in 1829, or a combination that fostered this imperative? Whatever the reason, my grandfather, who earned a modest income, could provide his five children with an excellent education: the boys attended the private Jesuit boarding school, Clongowes Wood College; two sons and one daughter went to university to study medicine; another daughter became an Ursuline nun, exemplifying a feature of family life that was not unusual at the time. The Catholic Church offered a refuge, along with societal approbation, for the offspring of the large families that inevitably bedecked a land in which procreation was deemed the only moral justification for copulatory pleasure. This symbiotic pretence allowed Rome to benefit from a steady stream of recruits to bolster its religious ranks, and the burden of large families throughout the nation was ameliorated.

The tribulations that faced my grandfather in fulfilling the educational ambitions he had for his children are evident in his application in 1908 for the position of 'Resident Magistrate for further promotion in the Royal Irish Constabulary'. This document also provides unique historical evidence of early policing policy in Ireland and the undercurrents of intrigue, violence and duplicity that would later bedevil the nation. Running to over twenty handwritten pages, this submission epitomizes the aspirations of a well-educated man struggling to educate his children in a poverty-stricken country.

After six years in the RIC, he obtained first place in an examination for the appointment of Assistant Clerk and was promoted to Sergeant and Clerk to the County Inspector. He was then appointed Head Confidential Clerk to Sir Owen Randal Slacke, who had charge of eight counties, and during his tenure in this capacity my grandfather dealt with the Tipperary Campaign, the south Kilkenny and Wexford agrarian wars, 'the prolonged Arklow Street preaching business', the Parnellite Elections in Waterford, Kilkenny and Carlow, all of which caused him such personal hardship 'that to recount it in any detail would fill a book'.

He was promoted to Head Constable in 1892 to take charge of Ballinrobe Station in County Mayo. During this time, he passed two Civil Service Examinations with distinction and in 1898 was promoted to District Inspector in charge of Tubbercurry Station in County Sligo. He records how, on his arrival there, Sir Andrew Reid, the Inspector General, alerted him to 'the grave condition of things within my bailiwick touching Illicit Distillation and requesting me, if possible, to diminish the evil and to report my progress in three months'. He appears to have gone diligently about his task.

After two years in Tubbercurry, he gave details of 'violent agitation' on the property of Captain Armstrong, necessitating 'day and night duty of a fatiguing character'; a dozen transport horses and fifty policemen had to be deployed to confront a crowd of some 700 agitators 'booing [and] band playing'. Numerous arrests were made, but my grandfather pointed out that 'it would be useless to institute proceedings at great public expense and that the trial would probably end in an acquittal'. As an alternative approach, he advocated having the parish priest speak to the offenders, and calm was restored. In acknowledgment of this innovative approach, he received a 'favourable record and £10'.

More serious crimes were dealt with as was fitting: 'A murder was committed near Athlone in 1901 and the offender absconded but I drew such a cordon around him that he was arrested on board a vessel in Dublin Bay and at Sligo Assizes in Dec. 1901 he was sentenced to 5 years' penal servitude.' In 1904 my grandfather was appointed with commendation to Thurles town (where my father was born in 1905), which 'had always been famed for highway robberies', and it was not long before 'a farmer named Gleeson was robbed outside the town of £20 or upwards'. The culprits were tried at the Cork Winter Assizes and sentenced to five years' penal servitude.

The patient wife who accompanied my grandfather on these custodial peregrinations around Ireland was Mary Josephine (*née* Aherne), who, to judge from the photographs of her marriage in Dublin in 1894, was a pretty woman and the pair made a handsome couple. She was from Waterford and presumably my grandfather met her when he was stationed there. They became parents of six children (one of whom died)[3] whose various birthplaces are testimony to the RIC policy of not allowing its superintendent officers to become too firmly established in one location; this approach was probably seen to be in the best interests of the safety of its personnel, or a wariness of familiarity in any one place being conducive to corrupt behaviour, or a combination of these considerations.

My Uncle Willie was a delightful man, who studied medicine and specialized in psychiatry. He was appointed to the Portrane Asylum (later St Ita's Hospital) on the northern outskirts of Dublin. My Aunt, Mai, who would later exert an influential role in my upbringing, studied at the National University of Ireland, where she graduated with a BA. She then taught in the Convent of Saint Dominic in Belfast, where she decided she had a vocation and entered the Sacred Heart Order at Mount Anville in Dublin. However, she was dismissed in disgrace for playing hockey with the schoolgirls – an activity deemed unbecoming of a postulant nun. She then entered the Ursuline nunnery in Waterford.

My other paternal aunt, Eveleen, was my godmother, a role that usually calls for affectionate indulgence – not that I recall her bestowing any especial fondness on me. She was a brilliant graduate of University College Dublin (UCD) and gained first place in a prize examination from the Richmond Asylum – a competition open to all Irish university students. She worked in general practice in the UK and returned home to distinguish herself in psychiatry.[4] Eveleen was appointed to St Brendan's Psychiatric Hospital in Grangegorman and was given a house on the North Circular Road adjoining the asylum.

I remained friendly with Aunt Eveleen until her death, but our relationship was strained by an incident that occurred in my final year of medicine in 1962. I was asked to appear on a 'careers' programme on Telefís Éireann, the newly fledged Irish television channel that had been launched in 1961. Why a medical student was invited to participate in a programme that purported to depict psychiatry as a career option is beyond me to this day. It may have been because Norman Moore, a psychiatrist, the 'expert' on the show, remembered me as a student who had shown interest in the history of St Patrick's Hospital, where Moore was the chief psychiatrist. The programme was chaired by the journalist Michael Viney.[5] The three of us were flashed across the nation in splendid black-and-white transmission with spots and dots all over the screen. During the discourse, which was being watched avidly by my entire family, including the psychiatrists (Aunt Eveleen and Uncle Willie), I expressed reservations about psychiatry as a career. I postulated that a close acquaintanceship with the mentally deranged could adversely affect practitioners of the speciality who might themselves become 'slightly touched' as a manifestation of a *folie à deux* phenomenon. The rank and file of my family, medical and non-medical, were (quite rightly) astounded by this preposterous appraisal of psychiatry.

Sometime after my grandfather's death, Eveleen invited Helena Moloney, the radical nationalist, feminist, actor and trade unionist, who had achieved notoriety during the Easter Rising in Dublin in 1916, to live with her. The friendship lasted until Helena Moloney's death in 1967.

Whereas I once basked in the pride of achievement in my maternal background, I now appreciate that the accomplishment of my paternal grandparents in raising a large family was comparable, albeit lacking the glamour of my maternal ancestry.

My maternal grandfather, Timothy Aloysius Smiddy (known affectionately by the family as 'Audo'), was born on 30 April 1875 in Kilbarry, County Cork. His mother, Honora Mahony (1853–1940) – a member of an esteemed Blarney family – had married William Smiddy, a wealthy victualler originally from Ballymacoda in east Cork, in 1872 at the age of nineteen. Books and treatises have been written about Audo. The most comprehensive biographical study of his career is *Envoy Extraordinary: Professor Smiddy of Cork* by Eda Sagarra, one of his granddaughters and my cousin.[6]

Audo's schooling was organized with the singular objective of making him a priest. He attended the Christian Brothers for primary education and was then enrolled in St Finbarr's Seminary in Farranferris, Cork. At sixteen, he matriculated at Queen's College in Cork (later to become University College Cork). The Bishop of Cloyne deemed him suitable for advancement, and he entered the renowned Grand Séminaire de Saint Sulpice in Issy-sur-Marne. He received his first tonsure in 1895 and transferred to Paris to study philosophy. However, his religious ambitions were surprisingly reversed when he departed the priesthood 'of his own free will' two years later and entered the Handelshochschule, the famed business school in Cologne. My mother told me this dramatic desertion from holy orders was because her mother, Lilian O'Connell (known to all as 'Muddie'), had 'snatched him from the celibate clutches of St Sulpice'.

To understand how this happened, it is necessary to appreciate the unusual education Muddie secured for herself in a time when women were allowed little freedom. Muddie, who came from a well-known Cork family, had been sent to Paris to study painting. She would have known Audo before his departure to Saint Sulpice, and she would have visited him in Paris, where it is likely that amorous sentiments led him to abandon the priesthood. Add a little tragedy to this love affair and the libretto could have been offered to Puccini. Audo's decision, while being a tribute to the love that bound them, must have caused the couple anguish. Audo would have had to resist formidable pressure from his superiors in Saint Sulpice, as well as from the clergy and his family in Cork. This termination of a laudable career in the priesthood would have been an unforgivable failure at a time when the appellation of being a 'spoilt priest' was justification for social ostracization. Muddie did not come out of the debacle unscathed: her exclusion from her mother's will was the family stamp of disapproval. Whatever the sequence of events and the emotional turmoil, my grandfather returned to Cork from Cologne in 1900 and married Muddie, the woman who had so enamoured him in Paris. They would have six children.[7]

Audo graduated from UCC with a BA in 1905 and an MA in 1907. He became Professor of Economics and Commerce at the College from 1903 to 1924 and was Dean of the Faculty of Commerce from 1909 to 1924. His growing reputation as an economist did not go unnoticed. He was invited to advise Michael Collins on the financial aspects of the Anglo-Irish Treaty, which was negotiated in London between October and December 1921. He was appointed Envoy of Dáil Éireann in Washington from 1922 to 1924 and subsequently Envoy Extraordinary and Minister Plenipotentiary of the Irish Free State from 1924 to 1929. This appointment is noteworthy in that it was Ireland's first formal diplomatic engagement with another country since gaining independence. It sought to strengthen the Free State's position by formally demonstrating independence from the United Kingdom. It also marked a significant development in Ireland's domestic affairs, being part of a campaign to discredit republican opposition. Audo travelled extensively across the US and Canada, speaking to societies and universities about his country's new political status among the free nations of the world and stressing the continuing economic development of the Irish Free State and the political stability in the country following the end of the civil war.[8]

The acme of Smiddy's tenure in Washington was the visit, in 1928, by the president of the executive council (in effect the prime minister), W.T. Cosgrave. The attention to advance publicity and to the recording of the many functions attended by Cosgrave is a credit to Audo's organizational capabilities. There are many informative photographs and films in the family papers in the Smiddy archive in UCD giving valuable visual insight into the social and political life of the period; these include remarkable film sequences highlighting Cosgrave's visit to North America and the celebrations marking the first aeroplane crossing of the Atlantic from east to west on 13 and 14 April 1928.

It is generally accepted that Audo was an influential figure in laying the foundation for the strong political and cultural bonds between the US and Ireland. In 1929 he was transferred from Washington to London to serve as High Commissioner of the new Irish Free State. He returned to Dublin shortly afterwards and advised the de Valera government on economic matters throughout the 1930s and 1940s.

I became close to Audo when he was appointed chairman and managing director of the Arklow Pottery from 1946 to 1959, an enterprise in need of the restructuring and efficient management he brought to it. When I obtained my driving licence at sixteen, he engaged me as chauffeur to drive him from his home in Dublin to Arklow, fifty miles away. While he worked in the factory, I walked the town and its coastline, observing the boats and the birdlife. Then, around midday, I would meet him for lunch in the sedate dining room of Hoyne's Hotel, where I can recall, not so much the cuisine, but the starched napkins that lay on the impeccably set tables. What did my grandfather and I talk about at those lunches? Did he inculcate principles in his teenage grandson? Alas, I have no recollection of the conversations that passed at these lunches, which I fear may have been an ordeal of duty for my grandfather. Encounters with Audo did little to establish a bond of friendship or love.

Of greater recollective impact, however, is the time I drove him to visit his three sisters, who had taken a house for the summer in Ballycotton, a small seaside hamlet in County Cork. Annie, Mollie and Maggie each wore velvet chokers and spoke in an appealing, old-fashioned idiom. The daily delicacy was a local speciality, 'drisheen', a pudding made from cow's or sheep's blood and innards. My hosts relished this epicurean treat, whereas I found it repellent. Picture me confined to the cottage staring out at the courtyard in an unrelenting downpour when I saw a mangy dog open the wire-meshed 'safe' containing the delicacy. I was faced with having to decide if I should dispel the dog, thereby saving the drisheen, or allow nature to take its course and be spared the nausea of ensuing dinners. I still suffer pangs of conscience when I remember my duplicity in sharing my hosts' grief when the felony was discovered.

In a biographical essay, Michael Kennedy alludes to an aspect of Audo's life that has been swept under the carpet.[9] He records how, as an Irish minister, Audo had to incur repeated hostility from some Irish Americans who attempted to bring aspects of his private life into the public domain. There were two incidents in Audo's family life that proved embarrassing for a high-ranking diplomat.

In 1927 his only son, Sarsfield, was arrested for bootlegging. *The Helena Independent* in Montana ran a headline declaring 'Sarsfield P. Smiddy, son of Diplomat is a Rum Runner'. The paper reported that on 26 April 1927, Sarsfield Smiddy, aged twenty-one, in the company of four friends who promptly absconded, was arrested 'while he was at the wheel of an automobile being brought across from Windsor to Detroit on a ferry boat … with 43 bottles of whisky … in the machine, most of it packed under the radiator'. The son of Professor Timothy A. Smiddy, Irish Free State Representative to the United States, languished in the county jail for an undisclosed period because his father refused to pay a bond of $1,500. Fortunately, he was acquitted of all charges in August of that year by the US Commissioner.

Another incident involved his daughter Pearl (better known as 'Binnie'). Audo's eldest daughters, Pearl and Cec, had accompanied him to Washington where they created a stir. Pearl was striking, with a vivacious personality that was not unduly influenced by the mores of her upbringing in Catholic Ireland. She fell in love with a count, Major Alfonso de los Reyes González Cardeñas of the Spanish army, who, in the family annals, emerges as a disreputable bigamist but whose life may merit reappraisal. His marriage to Pearl in 1928 was annulled by the Vatican, under guidance from Alfred O'Rahilly, one-time President of Cork University and later to take holy orders himself.[10]

Troublesome though these incidents must have been for Audo, neither would have impinged adversely on his political career. However, an amorous affair was another matter, given the mores of the time and the sanctimonious portrayal that Éamon de Valera and his episcopal ally, the Archbishop of Dublin, John Charles

McQuaid, were devising for the Free State. During his tenure in Washington, Smiddy fell in love with Mrs Agnes L. MacFeat, second secretary of the Irish Free State legation in Washington. and the first female foreign diplomat in this country. Many photographs of the period attest to the close bond that existed between them. Apart from the disapproval that this must have occasioned in the newly established foreign service in Dublin, the affair, understandably, caused my grandmother much anguish, and this makes sad reading in her correspondence. My mother mentioned this dalliance to me in hushed moments, but it is now known that there was one son of whom I know little, other than that he was an airline pilot.

Apart from his contribution to my chromosomes, my grandfather had little influence on my upbringing, unlike my grandmother Muddie, for whom I had great affection. I have two of her pictures, one a watercolour landscape, the other a copy of an oil portrait of an unknown mathematician from the Musée du Louvre by Ferdinand Bol. Muddie must have been a competent artist to have fulfilled the strict requirements to be permitted to copy the painting.[11] These paintings, and a portrait of her with her daughters Pearl and Cec leaning on each of her shoulders, are evidence of her skill, which fell victim to the financial and personal vicissitudes that marred her life. Had she been able to continue to study painting in Paris – rather than returning to Ireland to marry Audo Smiddy – she would have become an accomplished artist.

I spent many hours in Muddie's company at her numerous abodes, where she doted on me. I recall the gardens of Lansdowne House sweeping down to the Dodder, a flat on Merrion Road, and staying with her in Priory, Stillorgan, where her house looked out to fields and a small rivulet. I have warm memories of walking the East Pier in Dún Laoghaire with her, listening to her soft chatter, the content of which regretfully I forget. She suffered from depression during a sad, peripatetic existence, moving from one rented abode to another. She lived out her final years, after Audo's death, in Buswells Hotel and Hume Street Nursing Home, where I often visited her and where she died in her early nineties in 1969.

Her influence on the family has been underestimated. All I can do is pay a belated tribute to acknowledge with gratitude her presence in my life. I now appreciate how much she must have felt a sense of cultural deprivation in search of fulfilment.

My father, Gerard Thomas (referred to from here on as 'GT' as he was known in professional and social circles), dominates my reminiscences. Did he imbue in me the imperative to write, to record and to delve into times past? He had an unfulfilled wish to write, and I exhorted him to update his 'bible' of clinical medicine entitled *Systematic Case-taking: A Practical Guide to the Examination and Recording of Medical Cases for the Use of Medical Students* by Henry Lawrence McKisack, a volume I still possess.[12] GT was schooled firstly by the Christian Brothers in Synge Street, the mention of which provoked in him feelings of profound bitterness accompanied by expletives that would have made those men of the cloth cringe. He spent a short time in Terenure College and completed his education at Clongowes, where freedom from tyrannical punishment allowed him to concentrate on his studies. He entered the Royal College of Surgeons Ireland (RCSI) to study medicine and graduated in 1927. As a student in the Richmond Hospital, he obtained the Lyons Memorial Medal for proficiency in medicine. Immediately after qualifying, he left Ireland to join the Royal Air Force (RAF). This career choice was influenced most probably by the dearth of options to pursue a career in medicine in Ireland, whereas an appointment in the RAF offered secure employment, along with the opportunity to specialize. He was stationed with the 47th Squadron in Khartoum from 1927 to 1930, where he studied tropical diseases; this led to a Diploma in Public Health. GT seems to have enjoyed this period of his life – there were murmurings years later, when he reminisced over a ball of malt, of a liaison with a beautiful girl in the Sudan. To be sure, he cut a dashing figure and was often likened in looks to Charlie Chaplin, whose sense of the tragicomic in life greatly appealed to him.

On his return to Ireland, GT worked in Peamount Sanatorium, where he developed an interest in pulmonary tuberculosis, then the most serious health problem in the country. The illness killed about 10,000 people annually and left thousands of those who recovered debilitated by complications or the effects of well-intentioned but poorly tested efforts to cope with its pulmonary manifestations. To further his knowledge of the disease, GT studied radiology in the Royal Chest Hospital in London in the department of a fellow Irishman, Sir Peter Kerley. Kerley is remembered eponymously in medicine for his description of lines that become visible on a chest X-ray when heart failure is present: these lines are known to this day as Kerley Lines.[13]

Following his return to Dublin, GT was appointed physician to the Richmond Hospital in 1932, where the patients with tuberculosis were housed in wooden huts called 'horse boxes'. Many patients could recall brushing morning snow from their counterpanes. Two years later he was appointed physician to the City of Dublin Skin and Cancer Hospital, known as the Hume Street Hospital, and a year later he met my mother in this hospital where she was the resident house surgeon.

Her appointment had not been without opposition. The minutes of the Medical Board, dated 5 July 1935, record that Dr O'Donnell, seconded by Mr Coolican, proposed that Dr Muriel Smiddy be appointed as House Surgeon. The Board declined the recommendation on the grounds a lady house surgeon would be unacceptable to the governors and that this appointment was not in accordance with the terms of the advertisement. However, after much disagreement it withdrew its objection and, by November 1935, Dr Muriel Smiddy was firmly in office. However, in 1936 she resigned from her post; at the time female civil servants were required to resign their posts on marriage.

GT was elected a fellow of the Royal College of Physicians (RCPI) in 1937, and he achieved a national eminence as an expert in managing tuberculosis. In addition to his hospital appointments at the Richmond Hospital, St James's Hospital, Hume Street Hospital and Leopardstown Hospital, he had a large private practice at his home on Fitzwilliam Street. Without effective drugs against the tubercle bacillus, treatment measures were very empirical. Procedures such as thoracoplasty, in which a surgeon removes ribs to collapse and 'rest' the infected lung, and artificial pneumothorax, a procedure that likewise collapses the lung by the injection of air into the pleural cavity, were often of unproven efficacy in the days before clinical trials made it mandatory to test the benefit of such procedures.

GT loved poetry and music, especially opera. He was fascinated by the librettos that inspired composers, especially Puccini and Gounod. He was a keen cricketer, playing for Pembroke Cricket Club, and an avid follower of horse racing, if not always shrewd in his betting inclinations. Unfortunately, his career was blighted by alcoholism, which annulled ambition and dampened the promise of his earlier years. He published few papers and only one, a presentation to the Royal Academy of Medicine in 1937, had scientific merit. In this paper he presented a new technique for X-ray imaging of the lungs, known as bronchography, in which a radio-opaque dye is injected into the branches of the bronchial tubes to show their anatomy and to demonstrate any structural disease. This article predates descriptions of the technique in international journals. Failure to achieve scientific recognition can be attributed to its publication in an obscure Irish medical journal, which would not have reached the attention of international researchers.[14]

Of less importance, but of interest, nonetheless, was my father's inaugural address as President of the Biological Society of the RSCI in 1948 entitled 'Three Irish Pioneers of Medicine'.[15] GT invited Noël Browne, the Minister for Health, to respond to his address. Although a controversial politician, Browne was a logical choice in that he shared a desire to overcome the epidemic of tuberculosis by having instigated an ambitious building scheme to provide tuberculosis sanatoria throughout the country. Regrettably, however, when Browne took the podium to deliver his response, he failed to speak to the sentiments expressed by my father in his address, as would have been customary and mannerly, but unashamedly used the occasion to proffer his political agenda, much to the annoyance of the assembled guests. GT never forgave Browne for what he rightly saw as an ill-mannered lack of courtesy.

My father died on 27 December 1972, aged sixty-seven. His obituarist, Harry Counihan, who had been his junior physician for many years, acknowledged his pioneering work on tuberculosis in the era before antibiotic therapy, when surgical measures were the only alternative to lifestyle adjustment: 'He was one of the very few physicians who encouraged his surgical colleagues to operate on patients with pulmonary tuberculosis and other chest conditions where surgery is now taken for granted.' Interestingly, Counihan refers to an aspect of disappointment in my father's life that may have contributed to his escape from reality:

> Times changed, and the driving force of Noël Browne put into operation the reforms necessary to remove TB as the health problem. Gerry O'Brien applauded the changes, but his past efforts were ignored, and he was offered no recognition or recompense for his earlier services. It was a bitter blow and although it was accepted without a single word of complaint somehow the fire was dampened.[16]

My mother, Muriel Miriam (known as 'Moo'), was born in 1907. She went to school in London and then to Mount Anville Convent, after which she studied medicine in the RCSI, where she achieved top places in most examinations. She was awarded a gold medal in 1934 to celebrate the bicentenary of Mercer's Hospital, at which she was deemed the 'best House Physician Mercer's ever had'. Moo didn't practise medicine for long after marrying my father. I had always assumed this was so she could devote time to her family, but her departure from medicine may have been influenced by a court case in 1935. A surgeon in Mercer's Hospital, Seymour Heatly, was sued for 'assault and battery' by the parents of a boy who had died following the administration of chloroform by my mother. The court action was taken not because of the unfortunate outcome but because parental consent for the operation had not been obtained. Press cuttings recount that:

Dr. Muriel Smiddy gave evidence that in November 1934, she was on the staff of Mercer's Hospital as house physician, and Richard Holmes was a patient there suffering from goitre. On the 23rd she saw him in the operating theatre with an incision in his throat. A local anaesthetic had apparently been administered. The boy was restless, and the theatre staff were trying to quieten him by holding him down. He was kicking. Surgeon Wheatley [*sic*] was there and he directed her to give a general anaesthetic, and she administered chloroform. After a few drops the patient stopped breathing, and artificial respiration was tried for over half an hour, during which oxygen and carbon dioxide were administered, but the patient died.[17]

The devastating effect on a young doctor from a death due to treatment administered in good faith is now regarded as a calamitous experience in need of support, but such sensitivities would not have been recognized at the time of my mother's traumatic experience. She never spoke about this incident, which I uncovered in her papers after her death. The outcome of the legal action is unknown.

In my late teens my mother tended to lean on me for support as alcoholism overcame GT, who had distanced himself from all parental and household obligations. She did much to influence my childhood education and was always a staunch support in my medical career. She died from cancer in Monkstown Hospital in 1987.

If I was to define life as a gamble, it is fair to say I was dealt a pretty good hand. As a doctor I am often given cause to reflect on patients with a hopeless genetic history, whose future is inevitably one of damnation. Is it not this contrast of fortune and misfortune, of health and calamity, of decrepitude and vitality that constitutes the iniquitousness of the human condition?

2. *Childhood*

Children must be taught how to think, not what to think.
Margaret Mead. *Coming of Age in Samoa* (1973)

My parents had six children, of whom I was the eldest, to be followed by Berna, Hugh, Geraldine, Marie-Josephine and Mark. The creation of large families was inevitable in Catholic Ireland. Contraception was banned. Sex was solely for reproduction, and any deviation from this holy edict other than coitus interruptus wasn't permitted. The management of pregnancy in Dublin depended on social class. Affluent families had no truck with maternity hospitals, preferring the sedate security of private midwifery in nursing homes, of which there were many. I took my first glimpse of the world in one of these nursing homes, the Pembroke Street Nursing Home. (The more pertinently named Hatch Street Nursing Home would have been a quainter place of origin!)

I spent my early years trying to please my parents, which was difficult since I saw them fleetingly. Our upbringing was delegated to nannies and maids in the subterranean ambience of the basement of the Georgian house, Number 4, Fitzwilliam Street. My father saw his private patients on the first floor, where a waiting room, office and consulting room were reserved for this purpose. Every day the nannies wheeled my sister Berna and me to a private park thirty paces away. After a brief get-together with our parents in the evenings, we were left in the bedroom to play. Here I gazed out the window, my toy soldiers scattered on the floor, their wars over. On the wall was a postcard. I would look at it for hours, transported to another world. There were large oaks, their trunks bronze and their remaining leaves the colour of golden rust. Their arthritic roots clutched mounds of moss-carpeted earth. The setting sun cast a haze on the dale, etching the crisp and curling fallen leaves in detail. A stream flowed over rocks towards a distant city. In the foreground, a cottage nestled in the forest. This postcard has long since disappeared, but the memory of it opens the door to my nursery, where I can thread my way through the fallen soldiers and the bric-à-brac of childhood.

Fitzwilliam Street was awash with doctors. Just as Merrion Square a century earlier had been dubbed the 'valley of the shadow of death', so now Fitzwilliam Street was called the 'Harley Street of Dublin'.

The squares and parks of Dublin were our playgrounds. The Fitzwilliam Street Park was a friendly place, with tennis courts, a fountain and a roof-tiled hut with a bench for the nannies to gather while keeping a watchful eye on their flock. The tall wrought-iron railings were flanked by magnificent Georgian houses, their architecture erected for the nobility in what had once been the second city in the Empire. I spent hours in this oasis, where I had everything a child could need: security, trees to climb, pathways that seemed like boulevards, benches to loll on, and a fountain to drink from. Occasionally we went to Stephen's Green, where criminals were once hanged, but now boasting walks amidst statues and flowerbeds. My fascination as a child was the central lake with its ducks and swans. So many species of duck with dazzling colours. I marvelled then, and still do, at the clarity of colour when they emerge from the water, particularly the sheen of green on the heads of the mallards. And swans too – bigger and more threatening, but what whiteness!

My parents decided to move 'out of town'. I recall discussions later as to whether my father's practice had been affected adversely by this relocation, but whatever the reason, we moved not just to any old house but to the recently vacated German Legation at 58 Northumberland Road – the former HQ of the Nazi party in Ireland. During World War II, secret political, economic and military information was transmitted from here to Berlin until Éamon de Valera, under instruction from the American ambassador, ordered the seizure of the transmitter in December 1943. In the back garden, a mound of ashes bore testimony to the destruction of records. Heaven knows what information lurked in that one-time stronghold of Germanic administration.[1] Even allowing for my stature at that time – I was seven – the burn pile was mountainous. One day I probed the ashes with a trowel and a charred red cloth tied with string rolled out. When I undid it, something fell out. A bullet!

I was about to throw the cloth back into the ashes when I noticed the insignia that I would later learn was a swastika. Instead, I cleaned the flag and tacked a stick to one end. Days later, we assembled for our ritual daily walk. Our nanny emerged first with the enormous pram festooned with a sunshade, the edge furled with a corded pelmet. As the eldest, I took my place at the tail-end of the troupe, waving my flag. Just as we reached the gate there was a shout from an upstairs window. It was my father, livid with rage. Running down the steps, he took the flag from me and looking anxiously towards the road, stuffed it surreptitiously into his pocket.

Our walks from the former German HQ invariably took us to Herbert Park, its central lake crammed with ducks and swans. A pergola entwined in creeping greenery and a bandstand added to the beauty of the place. We spent so much time here that I even featured on the front page of *The Irish Times*, sailing my toy yacht on the lake with the headline 'The dawning of spring'.

Then there were the Zoological Gardens. My father was a member of the Royal Zoological Society of Ireland, so we were entitled to free access via a special turnstile that bypassed the many visitors.[2] So frequent were our visits that the keepers gave us menial jobs grooming the occupants, preparing their food and cleaning their habitats. The keeper of the reptile house knew all about snakes and guided us around his domain telling us which ones could kill with a single bite, and which were non-venomous. These he allowed us drape around our necks. The kindly elephant keeper, Jim Kenny, allowed us to groom Sarah the elephant and shovel her enormous turds into a barrow.

My father had a wonderful tale about Sarah. When in 1941 German aeroplanes dropped bombs on the North Strand of Dublin with loss of life, one bomb landed in the Phoenix Park beside the zoo. Sarah broke free from her pound in fright and disappeared. The keepers searched the zoo, but there was no sign of her. Jim Kenny was distraught. But then a vigilant keeper scanned the huge lake in the centre of the zoo and spotted the unmistakable nozzle of an elephantine trunk peeking just above the surface of the water, in the words of my father, 'like the periscope of a submarine'. There was Sarah, submerged safely beyond the reach of low-flying aircraft.[3]

I grew up in proximity to nurses, doctors and patients when my father brought me on his rounds. Hospitals were second homes to me, and I became friendly not only with the staff but with the patients who impressed me with their stoicism in the face of intolerable illnesses.

The City of Dublin Skin and Cancer Hospital, or Hume Street Hospital, as it was known, was where I was first brought into contact with sick people.[4] It was here that I learned to value health and become curious about the calamities that threaten life. Joan O'Sullivan was a most efficient matron, as was her sister, Tess O'Sullivan, matron in the nearby Portobello Nursing Home. I have a faint reminiscence of being introduced by Matron Tess O'Sullivan to a quaint, frail, stooped and kindly man, the artist Jack B. Yeats, who lived in the home during his later years. I was also friendly with the British pensioners in their blue uniforms walking the grounds of Leopardstown Park Hospital, chatting to me as they smoked their daily tobacco allowance.[5] Ballyroan Children's Refuge was a small hospital where children with 'consumption' were treated by nuns, one of whom lived in a railway carriage in a buttercupped field leading down to a stream.[6] I may have contracted tuberculosis on one of these visits.

The Richmond Hospital occupies a special place in my childhood memories.[7] Here I spent hours in the company of patients and staff while my father and his team treated the patients in his care. Sister McAnuff, the kindly matron of the Whitworth Hospital, was an imposing woman whose voice my father likened to 'slates falling in a quarry'. I noticed that friendly Smithy, one of the resident patients, who washed my father's and other consultants' cars, became bluer as he talked, and the cyanosis crept from his lips to his cheeks. I later learned these were the signs of advanced cor pulmonale when the diseased lungs fail to provide sufficient oxygenated blood to a failing heart. And there was another patient, Kitty, whose dwarfed figure, which was at first an embarrassment to me, soon became just one of the many manifestations of human illness that would accompany me throughout my life in medicine. She and I laughed in the rain that soaked us running from the tubercular huts to the main hospital. She laughed little in her sad life but was secure and cared for. Mr Fitzpatrick brought me for walks around the hospital grounds. I accepted his clip-clop gait as his idiosyncratic way of walking, rather than a peculiarity attracting the attention of passers-by. I would later learn that the slapping thud of Mr Fitzpatrick's feet on the pavement was a feature of advanced diabetic neuropathy.

Memories of these easy-going personalities endure.[8] These lowly souls, who sought no kindness from life other than to live in the hospital without fear of eviction, in return for which they allowed their peculiarities to be demonstrated to students – an absent knee jerk, a positive Rhomberg, an up-going toe, a hypertrophied tongue – gave much to a caring and efficient system of hospital care, but would not find comfort in the chaotic bureaucracy of healthcare today.

Moments with my parents left enduring impressions. I see my father in an armchair, grey-haired, sitting alone listening to the music playing from an enormous gramophone, covered by day with a duvet, wafting the strains of Rossini's *Cujus Animam*. The composition was, in my father's opinion, an inferior opus, but on this occasion any flaws in the *Stabat Mater* were dispelled by the exquisite voice of the Swedish tenor Jussi Björling. I tell him that the record has finished and needs changing. He asks if I understand the music. I don't know what he means but I put my arms around his neck and cry. He raises himself, and, holding me to him, restarts the record, and then, returning to the armchair, cries as I cling to him.

My father escaped his troubles and tribulations by immersing himself in poetry and allowing his spirit to soar with music. He loved opera and this obsession passed on to me. I read the librettos, the plots and intrigue of the great operas, but it was the pathos of the human voice – Björling, Galli-Curci, Ferrier, McCormack and Nash – that moved me most, often to tears. My father gave me my first taste of the theatrical beauty of opera. He brought me to his favourite opera, Gounod's *Faust*, at the Gaiety Theatre. I have never forgotten the feeling induced by the combination of pathos, music and theatre. With the poignant Apotheosis, my childish mind soared heavenwards, transported from the reality of the theatre to mystical realms, when suddenly a momentous thing happened. I still feel the shock as I crashed back to realism. There I was enraptured by this sublime trio when the celestial illusion was abruptly shattered, destroyed by the unmentionable proposition that evil had triumphed over good.

Another memory: my father is reading the line of a poem I have written in my copybook, 'the moon encircled in a misty halo of silver'. Could I have written that? Whatever it was, it impressed my father (for whom poetry was sublime in the hierarchy of art, taking precedence even over opera) and he reached for Walter de la Mare's poetry to read aloud to me.

Music often brings back moments of sadness. I see my mother standing at the black marble mantelpiece, her head on her arms, crying. A small brown Bakelite wireless with only two knobs is playing a tune: *Tra-la-la, twiddly-dee-dee, there's peace and goodwill*. I throw my cap and satchel aside and rush to her, putting my arms around her thighs and pleading to know what's wrong. It's her sinuses, she says, pointing to her face. But I know there's more to her sadness. She sits with me on the couch and asks about school, about my homework. Life between us would be perfect were it not for homework, maths in particular. I never learned my tables, and I can go only to M in the alphabet. My teachers tell my mother that I cannot succeed in life without tables. And without the entire alphabet, I am doomed.

Since the greater part of our childhood was spent in the basement watched over by a nanny or maid, it's hardly surprising that I can go back very far and conjure up minuscule details of our childhood surroundings. I just need one small detail to unlock a memory and moments come cascading down. Take the word 'Beeston' and suddenly there it is, a whole scene, as if yesterday. The kitchen with its bay window to the left, hearth ahead, pantry sharp right, tables, chairs, dresser, cupboards, cooker, fridge of antique ancestry, kitchen bric-à-brac. There was a small stove, called Beeston in raised lettering on its grey enamelled face, so endearing but out of proportion and inadequate for the needs of the room. Just to exhaust the Beeston fetish, there comes another scene in the basement that was abandoned in the evenings for the maids to entertain their friends. A cold, watery evening. I am late. Not wanting to ring the bell, I go to the window to tap on it. The shutters are ajar. I look in. They are in front of the hearth – the maid and her beau. He sits upright on a wooden kitchen chair facing the window. He has his hat on and a butt dangles from his mouth unlit, or rather extinguished from the want of pulling on it. No lights. Just the orange glow from the stove. Only van Ryn could do justice to the soft iridescent gold-brown softness cast upon the figures from the fire. One last touch – a half-drunk glass of stout on a stool within easy reach of the man's left hand. The froth clinging to the sides of the glass, a subsiding lattice of foam oozing slowly downwards into the black liquid. I creep away and later, much later, ring the bell.

Brittas Bay, a short distance from Dublin but far away in ambience and atmosphere, was where, for one month, my parents were ever-present and where we had time to express our love for them and they likewise. Brittas – a repository of memories:

dunes, sea, gorse, rabbits everywhere, until my father shot a family of them. Why? I never knew, nor perhaps did he – he was usually a kind man. The riverside shops of Staunton and Keogh, one on each side of the bridge, catering for all our wants, from food to buckets and spades. The village priest, still shell-shocked from World War II, delivering Sunday Mass to the hungover holiday multitude. The travelling players performing *The Murder in the Red Barn*, but above all 'Auf Wiedersehen' sung by a blonde-haired beauty, who melted my heart when I sat in the front row and she took my waving hand and pressed it to her cheek: the first waft of sexuality, an act of gratitude never to be forgotten.

The cove of the Rockfield Hotel. A dip in Jack's Hole (there's a place name for you). The long waits outside McDaniel's pub while my parents imbibed. Cricket with my father's friends, one named 'Little Sport', later to die by suicide. The horse and its owner, Gilbert, their scents indistinguishable from one another, seeing that they slept in the same barn. The big house on the hill where my father's friend and patient resided in summer, mistress of her coastal empire. Our beautiful nurse fainting during her pregnancy. My sister Berna, burning her feet in the embers of a fire. My father listening to the cricket test matches on the wireless. Music (was it the Palm Court Orchestra in the Grand Hotel?) floating through the bungalow. The gorse my brother set alight. Swimming in a blue sea and the dunes, ever-present, ever playful, sometimes threatening.

There was a story about three children and the dunes. Apparently, on a day of heavy rain the children tunnelled into them and nestled securely in their dry haven. But the dune collapsed, burying them. There was no sign of them save a painted bucket. Had they drowned without trace?

There were other holidays. A friend of my father who owned a farm in Wicklow persuaded him to send me there for a holiday. Here I learned how to milk cows, fend off bulls, be wary of geese. I observed a frisson between the resident maid and a brawny farmhand, which taught me much about life. The releasing fetish of this time is the word 'fuchsia'. Those rare days. The rising sun burnishing the landscape with a tint of orange brightening to golden-red. A cock crowing and the low moo of a cow reminding me I was not the only one stirring.

I went down the boreen, kicking a pebble in front of me, the collie at my heels. A rabbit fled, the collie in its trail. The deep red skyline paled, revealing the silhouettes of mountains in their furze-covered mantle. The geese left their pond to view the intruder and vent their ill-humour. A hedgehog curled up defensively as the collie sniffed its hide and gambolled off to the hawthorn hedgerow, which rose on one side to join with the fuchsia on the other. I opened the wooden gate to the field, tying it to a copper birch, which might have been planted for no other purpose. The collie and I soon rounded up the herd and we headed up the path, the cows, their udders bulging, cowpats breaking the silence, their tails swishing to dispel relentless flies. All was contentment. I wondered about my family in the city. How they were, what they were doing now. Gratitude welled up in me for my father, who had made the stay in the country possible. The cows entered the shed save one which I knew to have the least brains of all in the herd. It could never remember where to go. And yet I loved this cow, with its dappled-brown face, more than any of the others. I nudged it towards its stall, not wanting to make a show of its stupidity to the two farmhands who had entered the shed to begin the milking. I sat on a three-legged stool, a pail grasped between my legs as the men did, but I could never match the rhythm of their strong hands.

Later I went to help the farmhands mow the hay and sculpt it into stacks, which, would in time be transported to their destination on horse-drawn floats. I loved those days, the lunchtime breaks with steaming tea in tin mugs and coarse, ham-filled sandwiches, their charcoal-black crusts a delight in themselves. I didn't understand the lewd conversation of the farmhands, but I laughed when they did, so as not to betray my innocence. The smell of hay and horse all around and the sun beating down from the blue-blue sky.

Then it was shattered – my first lesson in the frailty of beauty, the underbelly of contentment. As I lay with the workmen in the shade of a tree, one of them suddenly grabbed me and undid my belt, saying: let's see what his little pisser is like, see if he will be a good stallion in time! His grimy hand mauled my genitals. But one of the younger men, who played the saxophone at night and worked as a labourer by day, told the older man to stop. Seeing the youth's clenched fists, he did. The saxophonist led me away, telling me not to be upset. I never forgot what he said next: 'Ignorance can never be forgiven.' I pondered these comforting words for years, which brought me solace after the assault. My regard for the saxophonist increased when I stumbled across Schiller in my reading, who put it differently, but only slightly: 'Against stupidity the very gods themselves contend in vain.' But, despite this, the beauty of that idyllic summer day had been despoiled.

Dublin was dotted with cinemas – the Capitol, the Metropole, the Carlton, and on Grafton Street, the Grafton and the Cameo, and the Stella Cinema, in Rathmines. Here a gaggle of children queued for what must have been hours, babbling away to one another in the little lane that ran aside of the cinema, intoxicated by the excitement of what was to come. The title of the film is long disremembered, but it was a western with the usual comings and goings, the horses – or 'hosses' as we preferred to call them – and the wagons, the hitching posts, the dust behind the hooves of the galloping horses through rock-strewn mountains covered in cacti. The hero and his betrothed surrounded by the evil one and his cronies, armed to the teeth. No one in the audience doubted that the hero and his heroine would survive and that good would triumph over evil. Picture then the shock when first the hero was shot and the same fate was meted out to the heroine.

We left the cinema in silence. In my bed late at night I cried at the perversity of what had been depicted on the screen, the victory of evil over good. All my teaching, the incessant indoctrination, had not even hinted that such might be possible. I banished the growing nucleus of a shameful thought, but it kept returning to haunt me night after night, that the pleasures of evil, not merely evil itself, might be more palatable than the complacent contentment of goodness that I had been led to believe was inviolate. And then came an even more frightening thought. Might my teachers be mistaken? Might not evil be the path rather than that of virtue?

And what of schooling? First there was Pembroke School, fondly known as 'Miss Meredith's' after Kathleen Meredith, who had founded it in 1929 at the junction of Baggot Street and Waterloo Road. It was small, with around fifty pupils, mostly girls. We sat in a room – twenty in a class – I remember nothing of what I was taught.

Two misdemeanours and one religious event left their mark. When we needed go to the toilet, we put up our hand and left the room to stand outside a door with a red or green block hanging on a hook to indicate whether the toilet was vacant or engaged. On one occasion I waited and waited only to realize that the last occupant had not reversed the sign. But it was too late. The inevitable happened. I returned to my desk, hoping the evidence would disappear. But the ploy didn't escape the ever-vigilant eye of my teacher. She paraded me in front of my peers as an example of male dirtiness.

The second incident occurred when a classmate crept into the back of the piano. His presence became apparent when the teacher decided to lead the class chorus to whatever rousing jingle she was banging out on the keys. For this crime, the culprit had to don a girl's uniform and stand in front of the class. He stood there, sobbing in red-faced shame. She stood there, flushed in anticipation of peer reaction to the pathetic sight snivelling in front of her. But she had miscalculated. The spectacle, which she assumed would have been seen as disgrace, was greeted by a collective derisory silence, as if, by some current of camaraderie, the class had been alerted, not to the humour, but to the nastiness she had created. Our silence puzzled and then angered her. Apart from these occasional indiscretions, which tend to secure survival in memory, the kindness of the headmistress, Miss Meredith herself, wafts across time as a persuasive influence.

My indoctrination in Catholicism began in this school. We learned the catechism and the ten commandments – many, like those forbidding adultery and murder, had no relevance to us at that age. How could we know what it meant to covet your neighbour's house, much less his wife? But we learned to recite them. Failure to do so would bar us from receiving our first communion, an event, our teachers reiterated, that would be the most important one, not only for us but for our proud parents. In preparation for this momentous occasion, elaborate rehearsals were conducted by Father Harley, who dispensed circular mock hosts cut from ice cream wafers, reiterating with authoritative emphasis that we were the privileged, who would soon receive the 'body of Christ' and that we must 'never' – 'never' being the climactic moment of all his exhortations – 'abuse this gift by sinning, or by not fasting before communion'. So, he droned on and on as he placed the mock host on our tongues, our faces upturned with a suitably reverential expression brought to fulfilment by closure of the eyes at the moment of reception and then slightly opened to maintain the sense of holiness while permitting sufficient misted vision for the walk back through the vigilant congregation to the appropriate pew without banging into a bench or trampling on the child in front. We were ecstatic in this miasma of wonder and mysticism. And when the big day came, I donned my new blazer and pinned a ribboned medal to the lapel to show the outside world that I was a first communicant. So, after weeks of instruction, we received the real host, the real body of Christ, from the hands of the very Reverend Bishop of Nara in St Mary's Church on Haddington Road, watched by our proud parents and our teachers, all uplifted by having been participants in securing another clutch of holy souls for Rome. Following the clerical ceremonials, I was taken by my parents to the Stephen's Green Club for lunch, where friends of my father pressed coins into my receptive hand.

Shortly afterwards, however, this religious milestone was sullied by a moment of irreverence. I was, at this age, most ardently devoted to Catholicism and would not have wished to do other than be seen as a subservient and pious adherent. In May 1947 Bishop Wall, Titular Bishop of Thasus, died and was laid out in full episcopal regalia in the presbytery on St Mary's Road to allow the parishioners to pay their respects. Being a devout Catholic, I decided to attend the procession and invited my Protestant friend from next door, who lived in a flat alone with his mother, to join me. Off we went to view the corpse.

As we joined the procession passing solemnly clockwise around the prone prelate, laid out on what looked like a dining-room table, I noticed a bizarre anatomical anomaly. The feet of the corpse were at an acute angle of more than ninety degrees to his legs, perhaps the result of a realignment of foot to limb by the morticians in their zeal to force the ornamental booties on him. The incongruity was ridiculously comical. I began to giggle and, of course, my companion joined in. Trapped in the encircling queue, we could not escape until a foul-humoured priest removed us. He then lodged a complaint with my parents, warning of worse to come from his superiors. The gravity of the incident was compounded by my deviant kinship with an illegitimate Protestant. I was taken to the episcopal headquarters to make apologies, with the assurance that I would behave as was befitting the son of a good Catholic doctor and, most importantly, I was made to vow that I would never again mingle with non- . Catholic children.

My home was not unduly religious, but one annual event has left an enduring episcopal impression. It goes back to Clongowes Wood College, where my father was educated. One of his classmates, Daniel O'Connell, became the Pope's astronomer in Castel Gandolfo in Rome.[9] Daniel believed that despite this venerable appointment, their schoolboy friendship bond should not be broken. Every summer, the Vatican prelate arrived for a dinner we all dreaded. The ritual rarely varied: at 6.30 pm, a black Citroën would glide to a halt outside 58 Northumberland Road. The Pope's astronomer would ascend the steps. A dinner ensued from which we, the children, were excluded. Then at 8 pm sharp, the Citroën would return with the Most Reverend Archbishop of Dublin, John Charles McQuaid.[10] We children were brought in to sit at a respectful distance in silence, imbibing the aura of holiness. The archbishop perched on the edge of a couch, sipping coffee; the pope's astronomer in an armchair on one side of the fire; my father on the other side with a palliative whiskey, sheltered by the pelmet of the chair cover, in reach of his furtive hand; my mother busily fussing over tea and coffee for the episcopal guests and finally we children had to kneel to kiss the huge pontifical ring. Bowing my head to the floor, I could see my reflection in his highly polished shoes that together with the frock coat made his presence one of sartorial elegance.

I progressed from Miss Meredith's School to St Conleth's on Clyde Road, established for the education of 'sons of Catholic gentlemen'. Bernard Sheppard founded the school in 1939 and was the headmaster.[11] He was a corpulent man dressed in brown, the waistcoat threatened by ash from an ever-present cigarette that defied gravity as he spun the weekly performance cards from the head of the classroom to each pupil with unerring accuracy – pink for the few high achievers, blue for the mediocre performers, and yellow for the minimum achievers, among whom I was sometimes numbered. Three successive yellow cards called for expulsion. Fortunately, I made blue-card status ahead of the dreaded condemnation. Sheppard meted out punishment on the palm of the hand with a leather strap (laced, we were told, with threepenny coins) and often sent me away in tears to the chorus from my peers 'dear Eoin, don't moan, don't moan'.

Illness intruded on my education. I was afflicted with tuberculosis – not a full-blown dose of consumption, but what was then known as a 'primary complex'. It came to light when I declined the pork steak my mother cooked every Sunday. No matter how monotonous this menu was, I looked forward to it with relish, so my refusal to eat was taken as a malevolent omen; sure enough, my father, the country's expert in tuberculosis, diagnosed the worst. Since it would have been inappropriate for my father to treat me, the Professor of Medicine at the RCSI, Leonard Abrahamson, known to his friends as 'The Abe', was called in to administer care. The Abe came each week to listen to my chest with his stethoscope, and his gentle kindness was made all the more memorable by the odour of cigar smoke wafting upwards as he ascended the stairs to my room, accompanied by my father. It was decreed that a protracted absence from school was necessary, whether for me to recuperate or because I might have been infectious to others, I am not sure. The former is more likely because primary tuberculosis is not usually infectious. Pleased though I was with this recommendation, my mother was determined that my schooling would not suffer.

First, she engaged a young man, Denis Donoghue, then studying at UCD, to act as my tutor for a few hours each week. He had a good sense of humour and loved poetry, Yeats being a favourite. One day my mother entered the 'school' room only to be faced with the spectacle of Denis Donoghue with his head swathed à la Lawrence of Arabia in the dust cover from the beloved gramophone, chasing his laughing charge around the room. On another occasion, we went to see a film in the Carlton Cinema. Running for the bus, I boarded ahead of Donoghue and, looking back, saw the tall, gaunt figure, who had an arm in a sling, trying to grasp the rail to hoist himself aboard the speeding vehicle. These memories are unlikely to have occupied the thoughts of this now-renowned scholar of English literature, but, for me, they are gentle and warm.[12]

The second measure taken by my mother to home-school me was to engage my Aunt Mai, who was unwell with an illness that defied diagnosis. My father arranged for her to undergo investigation in the private nursing home attached to St Vincent's Hospital on St Stephen's Green, where she became a resident for months. My mother now had a teacher with impeccable qualifications within walking distance. Mai had a BA and had held a scholastic appointment in the Convent of Saint Dominic in Belfast and, before her illness, was teaching in the Ursuline nunnery in Waterford. Twice weekly I plodded to Lower Leeson Street and up the granite steps of the nursing home to the room occupied by my aunt. She arranged a table and chair for me to sit and write at while she dictated the day's lesson from her bed. I remember maths, at which I remained utterly hopeless, and poetry – Yeats again – most of which I couldn't memorize, much to her chagrin. When the telephone rang one morning and my father told my mother that Mai had died suddenly in the very room where I sat for my lessons, I was relieved rather than saddened by this dismal news. I never recall seeing Aunt Mai out of bed. Perhaps this confinement contributed to her death; bed can be a dangerous place.

I recovered from tuberculosis and returned to St Conleth's, but it wasn't long before I was in serious trouble. A group comprising me, Dara Ó Lochlainn and John Gilmartin[13] passed St Bartholomew's on Clyde Road – an Anglican church. Gilmartin declared that a visit was overdue. He led us down the aisle chanting, 'Here come the true believers'. The vicar, hearing the hullabaloo, girded his cassock and rushed to challenge the infidels. This austere cleric then marched his three captives back to St Conleth's. Mr Sheppard, beholding the spectacle of the vicar with his hostages in full Conleth regalia of blazer and cap, realized the matter would challenge even his renowned diplomacy. Sacrilege had been perpetrated, the vicar explained; Catholics were banned in an Anglican church under pain of excommunication, as decreed by the Catholic Archbishop of Dublin, John Charles McQuaid. Then, adding flavour to an already potent stew, he probably threw in that the same episcopate was likely to be elevated to a cardinalship in Rome. The sentiments weren't lost on Mr Sheppard. He had no alternative but to expel us, asking the vicar that, in return, the matter be kept from the Bishop of Nara to prevent his boys facing the possibility of excommunication.

As a result, I was doomed to five years in the Catholic cauldron of St Vincent's College, Castleknock. The College, which had been founded by four young priests on the bedrock of Catholicism, with the motto 'Nos Autem In Nomine Domini' ('We, however, in the name of the Lord'), opened in 1835; its position at the forefront of Irish Catholic education was affirmed on 22 April 1900 when Queen Victoria visited the College.[14]

Memories of my time in Castleknock are punctuated by brief moments of happiness, but overall this period was one of darkness and misery, indoctrination and punishment, guilt and oppression. The first great pain was the estrangement from home and my parents. I had taken their love and presence for granted. Now I missed them. The pain of homesickness is like no other, save perhaps the misery of broken love. I lay awake at night in the dormitory of Saint Clet, named after a Vincentian priest who had been barbarously executed in China. His fate was of little relevance to me in coping with the 'wax' system – a modus operandi that had been honed since the foundation of the school. It was approved by the establishment and its priestly administration, most, if not all of whom, had been subjected to the same system in their schooldays, and who would attest that it had not caused them any harm. This procedure was initiated in my first week at Castleknock College.

Referring to us as 'scuts', the senior boys lined the new boys along the corridor and chose which scut was destined to be his personal 'wax' for the year. For the senior boy, this would be his last year at school and for the junior boy his first. The house captain – whose prowess on the rugby field earned this position – had the first choice. He would select according to his fancy, be it prettiness, hair colour, or whatever features most appealed to him. The vice-captain had second choice, and so on, until each of the fifteen prefects had chosen. I was selected by the vice-captain, perhaps because I was somewhat effeminate in appearance. Once the selection process was complete, it was the prefect's duty to inform the wax of his obligations, facilitated by another nicety in the system: prefects were permitted to stay up an hour later than the rest of the school. During this hour, each prefect could visit his wax safely tucked up in bed. 'The Crasher', as my protector was known (for his ability to remove anyone foolish enough to confront him head-on on the rugby pitch), outlined his role: 'You will be my wax. If you follow my rules, I'll look after you. If you don't, I'll beat the shit out of you. If anyone causes you trouble, I'll beat the shit out of him.' The Crasher visited nightly, regaling me in monotonous soliloquies about his prowess on the pitch as he munched whatever treats my parents had given me. Daily, I performed menial tasks, such as smearing dubbin all over his rugby boots so that mud on the studs wouldn't impede his burst for the line or diminish his ability to kick the oval ball into infinity.

The annual retreats were the prelude to each year of schooling. For three days, absolute silence was imposed, except for sermons and religious services – prayers, benediction, masses both high and low, confession and the reading of holy works imported in proselytizing pamphlets from the Catholic publishing emporium Veritas. These exegeses extolling martyrdom and sainthood with banality and righteousness could be purchased for a few pence. I consumed them fervently in my quest for eternal salvation.

I endured five retreats, but only one lives on in my memory, emblazoned so indelibly that I can recite the sermons verbatim to this day. A talented orator, a Redemptorist if memory serves, was drafted in, presumably with a brief to instil a sense of sin into the minds of a captive audience of would-be sinners.

'We will talk of the most grievous sin that any of YOU will be tempted to commit but I hope never will. YOU would be fools to do so, after the truths I will impart to you today.' The priest's stern face, with squinting eyes, stared at me. My God, I thought, he knows everything. The divine presence has alerted him to my filthy dreams, my foul thoughts:

> In America, a man and a woman were living in sin. Soon YOU will be their ages with their lustful spirits. But, unlike them, you will ALL be saved because God, in his infinite mercy, is giving you a chance to save your souls from the eternal heat of hell. Did I say ALL? No, not ALL! Some of you will NOT be saved.

The priest grew in stature and appeared to fill the church. 'The couple's car crashed in New York. The man was killed, but the woman survived, CRIPPLED, destined to live out the rest of her existence in PAIN. Her injuries were so disfiguring no man ever looked at her again.' The church was silent except for the rhythmic breathing of the white-faced boys. Next, he raised a trembling hand heavenwards and shouted:

> BUT her physical pain was nothing to the pain in her SOUL. Pray as she might; she could not find peace. And one day, as she prayed in a church for forgiveness, she felt a searing heat, and beside her on the pew at which her crippled form knelt, there appeared the burning imprint of a hand, the hand, yes, THE hand … of her dead boyfriend! Smouldering handprint! EVIDENCE of his banishment to the hottest of hells!

The priest paused to gain breath. He let the silence screech in our terror-struck minds. But this had nothing on the next oration, 'sinning with oneself', in which his rhetoric instilled even greater fear into his petrified audience. On this occasion the sermonizer was in fine fettle, entering the church with the air of expectancy that the consummate actor recognizes after a good first night:

> Yesterday we spoke of the evils of the flesh and the punishment that the Lord will inflict on any who follow the foolish course of short-lived pleasure. But bad though the evil sins of yesterday's couple were, there is as great an evil attracting and deserving a fate of eternal and everlasting suffering, and that is the sin you all can commit in the privacy of YOUR OWN BEDS.

He related how he was asked to give last rites to a dying young man, but it was TOO LATE! He was condemned to the fires of hell 'because he had had his chance of salvation but was foolish enough to squander it in his OWN BED. WILL YOU DO THE SAME?'

I showed an interest in books, and when I discovered a room into which hundreds of books had been thrown over many years, I asked the Dean of Studies, Father Walsh, if I could catalogue them. I was permitted to spend recreational time tidying and reading while my confrères walked the ridiculous 'track' that encircled an expanse of grass.[15] Senior boys walked clockwise and the rest anticlockwise (or perhaps it was the other way round) in groups of two or three, talking about, most probably, rugby. However, I recall one conversation about whether it had been within the bounds of purity for Grace Kelly to have indulged in mixed bathing in the film *The Bridges at Toko-Ri*, a censored version of which had been shown in the school cinema.

Some teachers tried to be innovative and to instil more than what was on the curriculum. Mr Brennan brought in his own Pye Black Box record player to enliven Shakespearean drama such as *Hamlet*; Father O'Flynn tried his best to get me to sing 'Loch Lomond' to secure a place for me in the annual opera; Mr Boylan made me aware of the artistic importance of perspective; and there was a carpentry teacher under whose instruction I made a card table and a desktop set of bookshelves, which I still have.

The school alerted me to the experience of religious mysticism, for which I am grateful. It wasn't so much the full high mass with Gregorian chant; it was benediction with the scent of incense that fired transference to an ethereal realm, where the senses were lulled in a haziness, that, sacrilegiously, I would come to liken in later life to post-coital bliss. All this happened in the serene chapel with its Madonna, where I served at mass. This was pre-Vatican II, with everything conducted in magical Latin.

Years of indoctrination lay ahead. If one believes in the Aristotelian maxim often attributed to the Jesuits: 'Give me the child until he is seven, and I will give you the man,' what hope is there if the clerics have you until you are eighteen? What I found so distasteful was the incessant inculcation of the righteousness of Catholicism and the hopelessness of those who espoused other beliefs. We were given no facts, figures, no comparative philosophy that might justify such intolerance. We Catholics belonged to the only religion that would see the face of God, and how fortunate we were to have been baptized into this fold. It was this hypocritical self-righteousness, so prevalent in the land I love, that alienated me from the Catholic religion and from all other faiths.

For whatever reason, I contrived to break rank, not with any sense of purpose, but with a desire to escape to what I intuitively felt had to be a freer, more tolerant existence. The opportunity arrived when I was prevented from sitting the matriculation exam in my fifth year because I had done less well in my second Intermediate Certificate exam than in my first. Not being allowed to sit the matriculation exam meant I was denied leaving school a year early to enter university.

This decision irked my father. In cahoots with the family dentist, Tim O'Looney, I espoused a passion for dentistry. O'Looney reasoned that I should pursue dentistry in the RCSI. This fitted well with my father's notion that 'doctors were thirteen to the dozen', whereas dentists were doing nicely. If a career in taxidermy had been offered as an alternative to school, I would have accepted it with enthusiasm. So, with an overwhelming sense of elation, through the rear window of a car I watched the creeper-clad school buildings and the playing fields of Castleknock College disappear.

My memories of Castleknock College will be at variance with those who prospered, went on to be successful and who dutifully consigned their male progeny to the same establishment. But not all of us benefited. So perhaps I can lay down a consideration for tolerance in childhood instruction: a resistance to inculcate the developing mind with doctrine and dogma; a realization that to do so can be to the detriment of maturation and expression; and that such manipulation of susceptible immaturity can lead to attitudes and actions that are detrimental to the individual and society.

II

3. *The Study of Medicine*

After five years of exile in Castleknock College, I was back in that patch of Dublin that accommodated an eclectic gathering of writers, painters and musicians. An artistic happening known as the 'Baggotonian movement' was later attributed to this myriad gathering, but for me, Baggotonia was a place with the intimacy of a village, where conversation gave sustenance to thought and expression that often lapsed into drunken banter.

My escape from Castleknock College came at a cost: I had no certificate and now had to make good this deficit by gaining admittance to the Royal College of Surgeons. This necessitated sitting an entrance exam for which my mother knew I would need tuition. Her prayers were answered in the form of an institution – if that is not the misnomer of misnomers – devoted to this singular purpose. MacDowell's Academy of Learning, at 33 York Street, specialized in preparing aspiring students for the entrance exam to the adjoining RCSI. No record attests to the existence of this institute, which enabled hundreds to qualify as doctors – time has almost swept away its alumni. The academy was owned by Mac, as we affectionately called its only teacher.

It was sited in one woebegone room in a decaying tenement house that was formerly a Georgian residence of splendour. A small electric fire emitted a flicker of heat. On rainy days an aroma of dampness emanated from the wet coats hanging on the backs of the wooden chairs. Ten or so students assembled daily to be instructed on the necessary subjects for the entrance exam. I can still remember Mac expounding on his beloved *Hamlet*, to which he gave his own interpretation spiced with innuendo: the stabbing of Polonius through the 'arras'.

My classmates were a mixed bunch. All, except a girl my age, were older, and many came from other lands. She was pursued with such intent by one of the mature foreign students that I had to spring to her aid and declare myself her brother. People with non-white skin were a novelty in Ireland then, and those who did grace the streets were almost certainly medical students.

'The Doc' from Galway was the eldest in the class. He had been attending the Academy for so long that he and Mac were bosom friends, often getting drunk together and jousting with their razor-sharp wit, to my delight and to the bafflement of the foreign students. The Doc earned his sobriquet by convincing his parents in Galway that he, their only son, was so close to qualification that their continuing financial support was justified. It was rumoured that he solicited funds from his village for a pair of amoebas – his mother, in granting the funds, enquired if they could be bred and thereby serve others in the cause of science. As time went on, the Doc's demands became more onerous. His father feared his son had lost his reason when he demanded the wherewithal for a pair of fallopian tubes. In complying, he urged his only son to be sure to realize their second-hand value over time. The Doc's other source of financial support was to gather a pub audience to hear his flamboyant tales, in return for which American tourists, who thought they had chanced upon a genuine leprechaun, plied him with stout. I can see him perched on a bar stool exclaiming, 'I was cooking my breakfast of eels and rashers, and when I turned my back on the pan to boil the tea, hadn't the bloody eel eaten the rasher!'

Mac often brought us to Roberts café where Josie, the waitress, reigned supreme. The place was awash with characters on whom history would later bestow the accolade of genius, but at the time they were just people, albeit eccentric ones.

I can still hear Mac asking the rain-soaked artist Kernoff, 'Jaysus, Harry, did you piss in your hat last night?'

I remember Mac with affection and respect, which is more than I can say for most of my teachers. Perhaps his liberal approach to education prepared me for the challenges ahead. Maybe he instilled in me a scepticism for authority. I learned how to study at MacDowell's. I devised a system that was very different from that in Castleknock. It was far from perfect – I still couldn't sift the essential from the irrelevant, the essence from the periphery – but I sat the entrance exam to the RCSI and succeeded.

I entered the College in September 1957 to start my pre-med year. I was seventeen, virginal, randy, obsessed by Catholic mores, which, if gainsaid, incurred the terror of hell and damnation. I was among the youngest in a class of a hundred students – the majority were in their late twenties or early thirties. Twenty or so students were Irish, with the rest from Africa (the Congo, Nigeria and what was then Rhodesia), the West Indies and a few from Asia. There was a remarkable cohort of mature students from Britain who, for a variety of reasons, could not live up to the academic standards of English medical schools. As for religion, there were Muslims, Buddhists, Jews, Hindus and Catholics. However, most students were atheistic and hedonistic. What a refreshing contrast to the stifling authoritarianism of Castleknock! This experience was as frightening as it was exciting. I found myself in what Ulick O'Connor once described as 'a university of life'. What O'Connor sensed in the College (where his brother Gary had been a medical student, and his father had been Professor of Pathology) was the ecumenical and cosmopolitan composition of its studentship. This heathen establishment surprisingly escaped the ever-vigilant eye of Archbishop McQuaid.

But I was still haunted by the priests of my childhood and surrounded by a subservient Irish society. Catholicism had claimed not only my soul but my persona. I was maimed intellectually and would have to cope with this infirmity for life. The repressive influence of Catholic schooling wasn't unique; my entire generation had been subjected to it. I questioned it and, in doing so, faced the consequences of emerging from the straitjacket of religion. In retrospect, I can see I was born at the wrong time; fifty years later and I would have been at ease with the contemporary pluralistic and liberal culture of Ireland.

Now I faced an existence for which I was unprepared. Routine and adherence to order was replaced by self-direction. I also had to take on a new role at home:

my mother began to rely on me in domestic matters as my father sank into alcoholism. Times were difficult financially because, his hospital appointments being few, he was reliant on his private practice, which was in decline. My mother tried valiantly to cope, and I accepted my unique role in the household as her adviser and confidant.

It would be years after I qualified before I discovered how inferior RCSI was compared to the medical schools of the universities. Whatever its deficiencies, however, it boasted a rich history. It had scarcely changed since it was granted a charter in 1784. The building was awash with busts and portraits of past luminaries. My favourite was of William Dease, a surgeon who, in demanding separation from 'that preposterous union with the company of barbers', had founded the College. His imposing statue, sculpted by Thomas Farrell, dominates the entrance hall. Among differing accounts of his death, one had particular appeal for me. Dease, who had been a member of the illegal Society of United Irishmen, on hearing of his impending arrest, committed suicide in his bath by severing his femoral artery and this was evident on the statue as a fissure along the course of the vessel. I knew (because my father had told me) that this was a historical impossibility since the statue wasn't sculpted until nearly a century after Dease's death.

Gradually I came to terms with the lectures, the lecturers, and my fellow students. I formed friendships, often with older class members who had experienced life elsewhere and were so much wiser. I resolved to learn all I could from them, and they sensed my need to grow up.

Life away from the lecture room and hospital wards was largely in the hands of the students. There was no organisational or financial assistance for student leisure activities from the College authorities, yet the diversity of activities was remarkable in sports and cultural entertainment. I played rugby with customary incompetence and attended debates at the Biological Society. I joined Milltown Golf Club, but having sent more balls onto the road than onto the green I put aside my clubs. I was no better at sailing. I crewed for Michael O'Rahilly (later to become a distinguished yachtsman and commodore of the National Yacht Club) in the only yacht owned by the sailing club of the RCSI, imaginatively named *Coryza*. Alas, the nautical excursion in Dún Laoghaire harbour ended in disaster when I dropped the centre board as we sailed into the path of the oncoming mailboat. Apart from the danger resulting from such incompetence, the poverty-stricken yacht club was landed with a substantial fine. After that, I substituted sailing upon the waves for the pleasure of swimming beneath them.

Student loyalty was to two public houses: the Toby Jug on South King Street and McDaid's on Harry Street. The Toby Jug was owned by Frank Swift and his wife, known simply as 'Mrs Swift'. The problems of life, women and exams were thrashed out in this emporium of eccentricity where students of law, medicine and politics met to talk and argue. When money ran short, as it always did, Frank would take a watch or ring against an advance to allow the stout and the conversation to keep flowing. His tavern exuded a unique ambience: the jostling throng calling for a drink; a group arguing in one corner, in another a bearded figure singing 'Four Wheels on My Wagon'; women held by men in familiar, confident embraces; and the master of the house filling glasses and shouting incessantly. Frank was squat with a massive paunch hanging pendulously like an apron over his bulging thighs. His neck, engulfed by the rising corpulence from beneath, had almost disappeared. But from his eyes – what warmth, what humour! 'Fucking Christ,' he shouted every few minutes, 'Fucking Christ!' A black mastiff, Moscow, followed him through the crowd and every time he roared 'Fucking Christ' the hound threw back its head and emitted a yowl that would have had a startling effect elsewhere but here passed unnoticed.

We frequented other pubs – Mooney's, Doheny and Nesbitt's, Toners, Neary's and Davy Byrne's to name a few – but the central pub for literary discourse was McDaid's, overseen by the gentle curate Paddy O'Brien, who controlled the unruly habitués and fretted that his student clientele might be led astray in the decadent company of older men.[1] We sometimes retreated to Bartley Dunne's beside Mercer's Hospital. This more cosmopolitan establishment, often referred to as 'Bartley Bums', was a place for serious drinking. Schnapps of 140 per cent Polish vodka and the bewitching voice of Yma Sumac unshackled the manacles of even the most conservative conscience. A fervent Catholic anaesthetist, downing his fourth schnapps, declared with passion that Joyce was right, 'obscene and filthy words enriched the whole business of fucking'.

My schoolfriend Kevin Duffy, who had the gentlest of personalities and a glorious sense of humour, accompanied me on my first venture out of Ireland. We took a rickety charter flight to Paris via London, where the high-heeled, tight-skirted ladies of Soho solicited the pleasures they had on offer. To us this was a new experience and very different to our brief visits to Dolly Fawcett's Café Continental on Dublin's Bolton Street, where ladies of the night mixed with lonely gentlemen in pursuit of solace, and where we looked on wishing that, like

Gogarty and Joyce in the days before these kips were banished to history, we could, as did they, share memories of the Hay Hotel:

> Where is Piano Mary say,
> Who dwelt where Hell's Gates leave the street,
> And all the tunes she used to play
> Along your spine beneath the sheet?
> She was a morsel passing sweet
> And warmer than the gates of hell
> Who tunes her now beneath the feet
> Go ask them at the Hay Hotel.[2]

In Paris, the naked statuary was a revelation to us coming from a land where de Valera had consigned paintings showing the bared female breast to the basement of our National Gallery lest the men of the nation (and, who knows, women too) might swoon when confronted with such indecencies. Had he not broadcast these sentiments unashamedly in 1943 by declaring that Ireland was to be a land where the 'fields and villages would be joyous with the sounds of industry, with the romping of sturdy children, the contest of athletic youths and the laughter of happy maidens, whose firesides would be forums for the wisdom of serene old age'?[3] But it was the Champs-Élysées that initiated the true unravelling of all priestly dogma for me. Here, standing with Duffy on '*la plus belle avenue du monde*', doubt rained down from the heavens. Had I not been told by my schoolteachers that Dublin could boast the 'widest main street in Europe' with its mighty O'Connell Street, named after the Liberator? The Champs-Élysées – measuring seventy metres wide was proof that this wasn't true. On that sunny day I vowed to examine the evidence underlying any statement of dogma, no matter how reverential or authoritative its source might be.

How did I not see through Catholicism earlier? I take solace in knowing that I was not alone. My friend John Banville also asked why we obeyed so meekly. He not only poses the question but provides the answer: 'Under a tyrannical regime – and the Ireland of those days was a spiritual tyranny – the populace becomes so cowed that it does the state's work for it voluntarily. And everyone knows, a people's own self-censorship is the kind that works best.[4]

Onwards through France we went, thumbing lifts and meeting people who, recognizing our impecuniosity and adventurous spirit, provided us with sustenance. At Perpignan we were penniless, yet proceeded on to sun-swept Tarragona. We returned to Paris destitute and put ourselves at the mercy of the Vincentian Fathers, who resided near the Luxembourg Gardens. After a brief interview, during which we begged for a small advance to allow us to return home with an assurance of payment once we reached parental security, we were despatched with a salutary admonishment that schooling in a Vincentian college did not extend to providing charitable support later in life. In desperation I turned to my father's educators, the Jesuits, whose headquarters were on avenue Hoche. I pointed out to a kindly Jesuit that my father had been educated at Clongowes Wood College, that he was an eminent physician in Dublin, and that he would repay any sum advanced as soon as his errant son reached home (adding no doubt that my father was a close friend of the Pope's astronomer in the Vatican). A modest advance allowed us not only to reach Liverpool, but to do so in comfort. Jesuitical kindness, maybe astuteness, when balanced against Vincentian parsimony and obduracy, reaffirmed my resolve to sever ties with my former educators.

Duffy succumbed, like other medical students, to the tempting offer to join Her Majesty's Royal Services – in his case, the Royal Navy – in exchange for his fees being paid along with a monthly stipend.[5] However, this Faustian pact required him to serve Her Majesty for three years after qualification. I contemplated the offer too but was saved by my insistence that I would serve only in Her Majesty's Royal Air Force. Whether this resolve originated from a childhood admiration for Biggles, or the heroic pilots of the Battle of Britain, or my father's sojourn with the RAF in Sudan, is unclear to me now. Fortunately, Her Majesty spared me by ruling that Irishmen were not acceptable as pilots, so I remained penniless but free.

I made many good friends throughout my years of study. Tom McDonald lived with his widowed mother in Sandymount. Our bond of friendship strengthened in our final year when we shared rooms in a former convent on the grounds of the Richmond Hospital. Our student rooms, known as 'Faith, Hope and Charity', were primitive, but the excitement of being on night call and involved in the management of acute illness put things in perspective, as did the night-time tea and toast with the nurses, and the promise of further solace. We lived for the moment rather than the occasion. Enjoyment had to be snatched whenever the opportunity arose, whether by preaching papal dialogue from the window to the inebriated denizens of the Liberties or making the perilous midnight climb to strike the clapper-less convent bell with an iron crowbar to add to the pealing bells of the city churches on New Year's Eve. Together Tom and I raised money for charitable causes, deducting a small percentage for an evening of relaxation after our altruistic endeavours. Our career paths would diverge: Tom, after serving in

Vietnam, settled in the Mayo Clinic, whereas I opted to return to Ireland after training in Britain.[6]

John Lynch, from Nenagh, became my cultural conscience, reminding me constantly that medicine should not displace the richness of literature. He was widely read, erudite in conversation and discriminating in thought, but he had difficulty passing the medical exams, which he often had to repeat. John and I spent much time together in Dublin's many bookshops, reading what we couldn't afford to buy.[7]

Lyn Greham Ronald Nash came to the College from Britain, having failed to meet the academic standard required by Barts medical school in London, although there were probably additional issues of subordination or misdemeanour. My first impressions of Nash were unfavourable: I found him to be a self-opinionated, prissily dressed, irritating Englishman who resented mixing with the 'peasantry of a backward, God-besotted country', as he once chose to depict his new homeland. And yet I grew ardently fond of this renegade, and he became one of my closest friends.[8]

Tommy Bouchier-Hayes came from a large family that lived on Upper Leeson Street. This mighty brood of thirteen children gave rise to a popular bon mot. His father, known simply as 'The Bouch', a well-known surgeon, on entering the Stephen's Green Club for a drink on his way home from Mercer's Hospital, greeted his friend, Fitzsimons, who owned much property, with the friendly aside 'And how's the squire of Baldoyle this evening?' to which Fitzsimons proffered: 'Very well, thank you, and how's the sire of Leeson Street?'

Tommy was well read, intellectually more inquisitive than me, taken to bouts of inconsolable love and, when lulled by alcohol and the strains of Beethoven's Pathétique Sonata, could become deeply emotional. When it came to study and examinations, Tommy had dallied for a year longer than necessary in the pre-med year – he was hopelessly disorganized, a weakness readily detected by his examiners, who had no option but to mark his dishevelled papers accordingly. Our symbiotic friendship was based on his need for order and guidance and mine for intellectual discourse. We traversed England in the summer of 1960 doing any menial job to pay off the debts to pawnshops and pubs incurred in the previous year and perhaps provide some financial security in the year ahead. We saw Albert Finney play *Luther* in Manchester, listened to The Beatles in the Cavern Club in Liverpool (oblivious of their impending fame), painted gasometers, picked cherry trees, drove forklifts in a brewery, charmed our way to Centre Court seats at Wimbledon, claimed the dole and served as waiters in Blackpool. Tommy gave running commentaries to bartenders, waiters, porters and drinkers – to anyone who would listen – on the Kennedy–Nixon presidential campaign, often incurring antagonistic reaction with his passionate belief that there should be a president of Irish descent in the White House. In Manchester, we chanced upon two delightful ladies who could not decide between a life devoted to nursing or the more lucrative preoccupation of being barmaids. One was Jewish, and she gave me her university scarf as a love token. I wore it for many years, and it would later serve to bring me into the company of Brendan Behan.[9]

In my first year, the so-called pre-med year, physics, chemistry and biology – euphemistically classified as 'science' – were subjects I had not studied at school. The Gaffney sisters lectured us in chemistry and physics. Ethna Gaffney I came to know and admire in later years but back then, like her sister Phyllis, she had to be convinced that I had the knowledge I knew I didn't possess or understand. I failed these exams but crept through in the autumn repeats after a summer of intense study.

Another teacher was John Henry Widdess, Professor of Biology. The only notes I still have from this time is my book of attendance at his practical demonstrations. Smells of formalin-fixed frogs and dogfish pour out when I open this manual. The hundred pages of illustrated notes present a detailed dissection of Scyliorhinus (the dogfish I caught in the Dodder river); the earthworm; the bedbug; the louse; the flea; the amoeba; the frog (caught in the garden and killed by passing a needle down its spine); microscopic examinations of skin, of blood cells and bacilli, including anthrax, diplococci, streptococci and staphylococci; and finally an examination of moulds, including penicillin – the harbinger of the antibiotic age. However, I wasn't always as attentive to Widdess as I should have been. I recall attempting once to enliven the evening lecture, when another student and I slipped down a trapdoor in the back row and, creeping under the floorboards, interrupted Widdess's delivery with windy sounds and knocks, to the amusement of the class. Widdess, aware that conditions beneath the floor of his theatre were tolerable for only a short time, moved to the back of the theatre where, standing on the trapdoor, he delivered in lugubrious tones one of his longest lectures on record.

Time cast me into many associations with Widdess. I am, at one juncture, his pupil, at another, his friend and later still, his doctor, who would care for him in his last illness. Additionally, I would edit a *Festschrift* to mark his contribution to medical history and finally be his obituarist in 1982.[10]

In my second year in RCSI, I came under the mantle of Frank Kane, the Professor of Physiology. His guidance influenced my apprenticeship and provided me with a methodology I used to good effect in future exams. I owe this man, who isn't celebrated in any archive, a remarkable debt of gratitude. Kane would set a mock exam in January when most of the class devoted little time to physiology. After the exam he brought each student into his office to discuss not so much the results, which were usually dismal, but how best to present our knowledge in future. Kane sat in an armchair by an open fire, which he kept stoked with coal from a scuttle. His desk, strewn with books and papers, was within reach as he welcomed me to sit so that we could both benefit from the hearth. 'O'Brien,' he said, looking through my flimsy exam paper, 'you have a meagre knowledge of physiology but a commendable talent for improvisation. If you were to blend this characteristic with a structured technique, who knows, you might yet qualify.' Kane went on to advise me to have compassion for the unfortunate examiner, to pity his plight, to remember that he might be ageing, that his sight might be failing and that it was a foolish student who expected him to read through pages of nonsense seeking the rare gem of knowledge therein:

> Remember, O'Brien, that the examiner may have the dyspeptic task of facing a hundred essay papers on a sunny June afternoon after a pleasant lunch, which he will now round off with a ball of malt. *Ease* his task, O'Brien, *help* him to give you a good mark by structuring your answers. Tell him at the outset that you propose to answer the question under the headings one, two, three. In this way, the examiner doesn't have to read all the nonsense you write; he just marks you up for the knowledge you have and subtracts for that which you obviously don't possess.

There were other lessons to be learned from this wise man. He abhorred note-taking during his lectures, but students did not heed his advice: in their opinion, he was eccentric. One day, during a lecture on Starling's Law, Kane interspersed his scientific narrative with a comment that went something like: 'The force of contraction of the heart muscle made the rats die, and the stench was awful.' Then he paused and asked a Trinidadian beauty with an ebony curvaceousness that could be very distracting, to read her notes, which, like so many in the class, contained his exact words.

I was among the last students to be lectured on anatomy by the enigmatic and much revered Tom Garry. In the Anatomy Room, sitting around a cadaver, we watched Garry hold up one colourless strand of tissue after another to demonstrate the importance of knowing the relationship of every blood vessel to the organs we might later remove if we became surgeons. For those with aspirations to be orthopaedic surgeons, Garry stressed the significance of knowing the point of *origin* and *insertion* of the muscles in the body that governed motion, a topic that allowed him to indulge in racy innuendo by stating that the longest muscle in the body had its origin in Grafton Street and its insertion in the Phoenix Park. We didn't know then of his fame or reputation, which he himself held in high regard, claiming that the only reliable authorities on the anatomical structure of the human body were God and he and that if truth be known, he was the better versed. To meet the criteria of the Fellowship Examination in Surgery, which demanded an intimate knowledge of human anatomy, doctors from around the world attended Garry's grind, as he acknowledged in his epitaph:

> From the north pole to the south, through the
> wilderness of the eternally white plains of Siberia,
> the darkest bush of Africa, the southern seas;
> from the venerably aged coast of China, through
> the old continent, to the beaches of the sometimes too
> new continent, where the name of Jesus Christ is unknown;
> the name of Tom Garry is a household word.[11]

In my final year and Garry's last year of life I was saddened to see this lonely man, who I knew lived in solitude and apparent contentment in his tenement room where he delivered his grinds, sipping a glass of stout in the upstairs bar of Neary's. More out of kindness than inquisitiveness, I asked if I could join him. We discussed his long-awaited book of anatomy, which it was rumoured would be superior to Gray's classical monograph. He assured me it was nearing completion but doubted if it would see the light of day. Unfortunately, he was right – the tome perished in a fire that consumed the contents of his hovel on York Street.

The anatomy room was a new experience. The naked, shrivelled bodies of men and women lay on tables, having been temporarily released from tanks to recommence dissection on whatever organ or vessel had been the focus of tuition the previous day. The atmosphere was laden with the pungent, pickle-vinegar smell of formalin, a unique aroma that I will always associate with the tanks of the dead and which I didn't find unpleasant. Here we carried out respectful bodyside learning from demonstrators, while the Professor of Anatomy, Gilbert Marshall Irvine, positioned in an office high on a wrought-iron balcony, kept a watchful eye. We dissected every part of the human body. We learnt the relationship of nerve to vein and artery, muscle to bone, heart to lung in the thoracic cavity; how the abdominal organs jostled for position within the confines of a space that allowed a palpating hand to detect mischief within one or other organ; the majestic pathways that permitted the transmission of complex messages from the brain via the spinal cord to the most distal extremity – in short, the magnificence of the human form.

In the 1960s students of medicine and dentistry sat the same examinations before parting company. The former would spend the next three years attached to the teaching hospitals of the College, and the latter would transfer to the Dental Hospital on Lincoln Place. I spent three months receiving tedious instruction on the materials used in dentistry, such as moulding wire around nails on blocks of wood. I sat one examination – Dental Metallurgy, in which I achieved the distinction of being awarded zero. This was a disappointment. I expected my answer to 'discuss the uses of wire in dentistry' to be given at least one mark for my humorous assessment that had within it a truism. Having rewired the complex system of bells that extended from room to room in my family home, I applied this knowledge to a treatise (with diagrams) to show how dependent the dentist was on the doorbell that announced a patient's arrival. Without this contrivance, I concluded, the dentist would be denied a living. Following this dismal exam result, my father had to admit I wasn't suited to dentistry, and so, three months adrift of my colleagues, I turned to medicine.

The engrossing intensity of clinical medicine would change my life profoundly. It also restored purpose to my existence. I now embarked on three happy years as a 'clinical clerk', walking the wards of the Richmond Hospital, where I rotated among the physicians and surgeons. There was much work to be done, and clerks were an indispensable part of the system. I was tutored in the art of recording a patient's history. I learned to take blood and how to examine patients and elicit the clinical signs leading to a diagnosis.[12]

The bedside clinic constituted a unique educational process whereby the normal duality of communicating knowledge between a teacher and a student was enhanced by the presence of an essential interloper – the patient. Indeed, some patients who boasted the manifestations of chronic illness, such as diabetic neuropathy, valvular heart disease or chronic bronchitis and emphysema, became so proficient in the ritual that the bedside clinic became a piece of finely rehearsed theatre in which the patient would react on cue from the clinician, not only to fulfil the necessary educational purpose of the tripartite exchange, but to do so with wit and panache.

The teacher introduced the patient to the twenty or so students clustered around the bed. One would be selected to interrogate the patient according to a methodology aimed to reveal the presenting complaint, any previous conditions, the family history and behavioural factors that might influence the patient's health. Another student was selected to examine the patient according to a procedure that would reveal abnormalities in the nervous, gastro-intestinal, respiratory and circulatory systems. Discussion would then focus on how these findings, and the history, might lead to a list of provisional diagnoses. A student would then be called upon to enumerate the investigations that might confirm the ultimate diagnosis, and finally a student would be questioned on how the patient should be treated. These bedside encounters were not without moments of pathos when the student, patient and teacher simultaneously became aware of the pain of the human condition. Some encounters were memorable as lessons of my clinical incompetence. At a bedside clinic on a patient recovering from a heart attack, Harry Counihan, the consultant, gave me a sphygmomanometer and asked me to measure the patient's blood pressure. I had never done this before – such a menial task was delegated to nurses. I revealed my ineptitude by not only having difficulty opening the sphygmomanometer box but also by not knowing how or where to wrap the cuff. I sometimes wonder if this inauspicious introduction to the vagaries of blood-pressure measurement had any bearing on my dedication to the scientific nuances of the technique in my future research.

After being tutored in medical illnesses, I rotated to the surgical side of the hospital, where the same process was repeated. In this way, some excellent teachers taught me the essentials of diagnosis, management and treatment over three years, during which my progress was assessed by examinations at regular intervals. I also spent time in the casualty department, assisting senior colleagues in the emergency treatment of patients. Since the Richmond Hospital was the national centre for neurosurgery, I became familiar with all forms of neurological disease. Knowing about the multiple pathways along which nerve impulses travel between the brain and the receptors fascinated and terrified me. Brendan McEntee, a neurologist par excellence, was crippled by childhood poliomyelitis, but his disability endeared him to his patients whose trust and confidence were absolute. Tucking his walking cane under the mattress, he perched – there was no other word for it – his fragile frame alongside the patient. He interrogated them in gentle, compelling tones and then examined them with ease: a tap of the reflex hammer to elect an increased ankle or wrist jerk; a finger pointing to a fine tremor; a moving finger to be followed by nystagmoid eyes; and finally, the integration of the patient's symptoms with the clinical peculiarities to form a diagnosis. These were magical performances, the skill of which became apparent when I tried so inadequately to emulate them.

The consequences of neurological calamities terrified me. I recall a beautiful young girl who had had a subarachnoid haemorrhage. A lumbar puncture was performed to diagnose the presence of blood in ordinarily clear spinal fluid. The demonstration was flawless. But the spinal fluid showed blood, confirming the need to refer the girl to the neurosurgeons so they could obliterate the aneurysm that had caused the bleed. However, shortly after the lumbar puncture, the girl lost consciousness and died. A dreaded complication known as 'coning' had occurred, whereby the lowering of pressure in the spinal canal from the lumbar puncture enabled the raised pressure in her skull, resulting from the haemorrhage, to push part of her brain through the narrow opening in the skull. We students, who had only just spoken with the girl, were devastated by this sudden and cruel ending of her life.

Another haunting memory was of an old man I clerked. I noticed that his left eye was inert and unreactive but in the right the pupil quivered, dilating and contracting, but only slightly. I realized he was trying frantically to communicate. He had what is now known as the locked-in syndrome.[13] I alerted the nurses and his physician that whatever conversation took place around his bed should be gentle and take account of the fact that he understood. I tried to persuade the nurses to give him drugs to relieve his suffering and stop the pupil from convulsing, as it did when he was distressed, but such kindnesses were not condoned.

Another time, the neurosurgeon Paddy Carey presented a man my age whose spinal cord had been severed and whose body had become a useless appendage to the impulses pouring from his frenzied brain. Immediately I saw the enormity of his suffering: the wasting limbs; the flattened buttocks; the reddening heels; the futile penile shaft; the thoracic cage that functioned only with mechanical assistance; the wild and furtive eyes that could make no protest; the mouth full of tubes from which there articulated, nonetheless, a message of damnation; the dark, dark hair; the handsome brow. It was too much. I had to be lifted from the floor and laid on a bench in a tiled corridor beneath the bronze relief of one named William Thompson. A nurse brought me water and tenderly wiped my dank brow.

Another painful memory endures. She was perhaps thirty, but she looked ten years older, such was her suffering. She clasped the bedclothes with her fists as paroxysms of pain wracked her wasted body and tears flowed from her still-beautiful eyes. I was aware of the teacher droning on and on, indifferent to her anguish, oblivious that in her suppressed cries might be the scream for dignity as he probed and dug his hand into her abdomen and then exposed her shrivelled breasts, pontificating, as he did so, to the mostly indifferent gallery. I didn't feel bitterness toward my mentor or despise him. I felt pity for him, tinged with scorn. Later I went back to the woman and asked if she needed anything. She was no longer in pain; they had given her something. Why, I wondered, did they keep her alive? She did not want to die yet, she said. The pain I'd witnessed was nothing to the other pain. 'Other pain?' I cried, rising from the bedside in horror, 'Where's the *other* pain?' 'There,' she replied, pointing to her head and then to her heart. She told me about her cancer, her dead husband and three young children with no one to look after them. A day later I felt strong enough to revisit this sad woman, but she was gone.

The spectrum of diseases was different then to what a student faces now. If the drugs available to treat illness were primitive by today's standards, the surgical options for treating cardiac disease today couldn't have been imagined in the 1950s. The cardiac manifestations of rheumatic fever accounted for much of the illnesses in the medical wards whereas today rheumatic fever is rare in Irish hospitals. To pass the final exams, I had to know that rheumatic fever (caused by the streptococcus bacteria) announced its presence in the joints as acute arthritis. It caused a plethora of symptoms and abnormalities in many tissues and organs. For example, one patient might develop skin lesions; another might develop rapid, uncoordinated jerking movements affecting the face, hands and feet (known as Sydenham's chorea or Saint Vitus' dance) due to the damaging effect of the bacteria on the brain;[14] but the heart bore the brunt of the assault. Acute rheumatic fever could also present as an immediate life threat. When the lining pocket around the heart becomes inflamed, a creaking rub is audible with the stethoscope. The intense chest pain might be relieved only by leaning forward in the sitting position to separate the inflamed surfaces of the pericardial sac. If the fluid from the inflamed surfaces becomes excessive, the heart is compressed and, in severe cases, is unable to continue pumping, causing a medical emergency known as cardiac tamponade. I recall a young woman being brought into the casualty department of the Richmond Hospital with extreme breathlessness caused by tamponade, which was dramatically relieved when I inserted a needle into the pericardial space to drain the accumulated fluid.

Cardiac manifestations were all the more challenging to diagnose and treat because the presenting abnormalities, though initially slight, would progress over the years. The heart valves were attacked with either thickening (stenosis) or floppiness of the supporting cords, causing leaking (incompetence), which interfered with their primary function by either preventing blood from going forward through the stenosed valve or by permitting it to flow back, or regurgitate, through the incompetent valve. These abnormalities produced murmurs in the heart at various parts of the cardiac cycle that could, with training, be detected with a stethoscope. Failure to auscultate these sounds augured badly for the final exams.

My father told me the interesting history of the stethoscope, which, although now relegated to being little more than a talisman of medicine, was an indispensable diagnostic instrument in my student days. Technologies such as magnetic resonance imaging (MRI) and echocardiography have rendered the subtle abnormalities of sound from a diseased heart superfluous. The denigration of the stethoscope is apparent in how the instrument is now 'worn'; in my student days it hung from the neck within easy reach of the wearer's ears, whereas today it is draped across the back of the neck to denote a hierarchical entitlement. Nonetheless, the stethoscope, more than any other instrument, has provided the diagnostic information to guide treatment in countless patients throughout the world.

The use of the stethoscope in Britain and Ireland can be attributed to an Irish student, William Stokes. When studying medicine in Edinburgh in 1825, Stokes was so impressed with a publication by René Théophile Hyacinthe Laënnec – a physician in the Necker Hospital in Paris – that he wrote a treatise on it.[15] The stethoscope underwent many iterations before reaching its present form. Before Laënnec's publication, sounds in the lungs and heart were listened to by placing the ear directly against the chest, a technique known as immediate auscultation. Wishing to auscultate the chest of a young girl but being too embarrassed to place his ear on her chest, Laënnec remembered that if the ear is placed against one end of a wooden beam, the scratch of a pin at the other end is distinctly audible. He rolled a sheet of paper into a tube and placed one end over the girl's chest and his ear to the other and was elated to hear the heart beating with greater clearness than he ever had with immediate auscultation. He immediately saw that this might become an indispensable method for studying not only the heart but any organs that produced sounds and he went on to develop various types of monaural stethoscopes.

The new instrument was adopted by Stokes's Irish classmate, Dominic Corrigan, who used it to listen to the heart of a patient with rheumatic valvular disease and aortic regurgitation, known to this day as 'Corrigan's disease'.[16] Corrigan, in keeping with the Victorian spirit, liked to visit hospitals in the major cities of Europe. On one such a visit to a Parisian hospital, one of the French physicians proclaimed a patient to be suffering from '*maladie de Corrigan*' and, remembering the name of his guest, asked him if he knew Corrigan of Dublin, to which Corrigan promptly replied, '*C'est moi, monsieur.*' He was led to the lecture theatre and presented with acclaim to the staff and students. In America, writers began referring to the characteristic pulse as 'Corrigan's pulse', and because the pulse bore a resemblance to the sensation given by the popular Victorian toy known as the 'water-hammer', it was often referred to as the 'water-hammer pulse'.[17]

My father tutored me in the use of the stethoscope and trained me to recognize the all-too-ominous signs of ravaging pulmonary tuberculosis that had blighted Ireland for over a century. With his stethoscope, he mimicked the sounds he heard and interpreted them for me. Many of these descriptive terms had a musical allure – sibilant and sonorous rhonchi, coarse and fine crepitations, whispering pectoriloquy, and aegophony. Contemporary medical students and doctors would not know the meaning of this descriptive language because the underlying pathology that gave them meaning no longer exists, and the auscultatory skill to detect such auditory phenomena has duly waned. My father showed me how to induce an artificial pneumothorax by introducing air into the pleural cavity to 'rest' the diseased lung. Then, in an adjoining room, he had his primitive X-ray apparatus where he would screen the patient's chest and heart, and then take an X-ray film that I would develop for him. His upper body was protected from radiation by a lead apron but the scatter of radiation to his feet was considerable, as evidenced by my mother entering into a discount arrangement with a cobbler to repair and eventually replace my father's decaying footwear.

In the late 1950s, the drugs available for treating disease were limited. There had been few advances in pharmacology other than the recent introduction of antibiotics. The lack of therapeutic options is illustrated by a gentle patient named James, who was allocated to me as a student for daily clerking. James had become increasingly short of breath on exertion over several years. At the time of his hospital admission, he became breathless at night if he didn't sit upright, preferably in a chair. In addition, he developed swelling of his ankles, which spread to his thighs and abdomen. Finally, his entire scrotal area became painfully swollen. These symptoms and clinical manifestations constituted the diagnosis of 'dropsy'. James was unresponsive to injections of mersalyl, the recently introduced diuretic drug. In desperation, a set of Southey's tubes were unearthed in the hospital pharmacy. Southey's tubes had once been widely used to drain off excessive fluid in patients with dropsy. Fine-calibre silver or brass cannulas were inserted into fluid-swollen legs and, when attached to rubber tubes, could drain as much as six litres of fluid in twenty-four hours, giving relief to patients.[18] On one of my morning visits to assess James's progress, I noticed that, although he had obtained relief from the removal of fluid with the Southey tubes and could now sleep upright at night in a chair without fear of suffocating, he had developed another troubling discomfort. His feet, resting in basins into which the fluid from the Southey tubes drained, had become excoriated and painfully tender. I attached plastic bags to each Southey tube which, when filled, could be replaced and his feet were no longer immersed in the drained fluid. This simple expedient removed one affliction from the terminal suffering of this stoic patient. This vignette, which emphasizes the relevance of the empirical principles in medicine, also illustrates how little medicine had advanced in the century that separated me, as a student, in the 1950s from Corrigan, the physician, in the 1840s; it also serves as a comparative landmark against which the revolutionary procedures in cardiac treatment over the next fifty years can be assessed.

As a student, I had two other investigations to assist me in the diagnosis of cardiac illnesses. The ECG permitted me to determine the size of the heart (usually enlarged in patients with rheumatic heart disease), the rhythm and rate of the heart (often rapid and irregular because of atrial fibrillation) and any damage to the heart muscle by the narrowing of the coronary arteries. I was introduced to electrocardiography in Hume Street Hospital when I assisted Nell Sheridan, the radiographer, to record the ECG with a device my father purchased for the hospital. Recording an ECG was then an elaborate procedure. The electrodes were large and required the liberal use of jelly to make contact with the skin. The ECG was recorded on film, which then had to be processed by 'developing and fixing' into a reasonable printed record.[19] The second tool I used was radiology to examine the movement of the heart by screening it in action. I could view X-rays of the heart and lungs to show me the size of the heart, and the presence of any fluid in the lungs caused by heart failure.

My long experience as a doctor allows me to appraise a century of medical progress by comparing the remedial poverty of 'then' with the therapeutic abundance of 'now'. For example, I could treat the cause of rheumatic valvular disease, even hope to eradicate it, and I could alleviate the symptoms of a failing heart with diuretics, but I could do little for patients with severe valvular damage or for those suffering from heart attacks, whose mortality was high. But this was about to change. As I neared qualification, two major developments were to change the progress of patients with cardiac disease: the first was the surgical replacement of diseased valves and the second was the advent of techniques to open occluded coronary arteries. Ultimately, transplanting a heart would become a commonplace procedure. This is remarkable when we remember that to operate on the heart was seen as a violation of sacred function; the myth was shattered when surgeons began to view the heart as being amenable to intervention like any other organ.

The first major advance was being able to repair valves distorted by rheumatic fever. The first successful operation using a heart-lung machine in 1953 allowed surgeons to perform complicated procedures on a bloodless open heart with enough time to correct structural abnormalities. However, although repairing diseased valves improved the quality of life for patients, the introduction of prosthetic valves in 1961 would benefit many thousands of patients worldwide with valvular disease. In recent years, corrective manipulations of the valves have passed from the surgeon to the interventional cardiologist, who can now correct valvular abnormalities from the femoral vein, thereby avoiding the need for open-heart surgery altogether. This half-century of dramatic achievement has been accompanied by technological innovations leading to implantable pacemakers and defibrillators to treat abnormalities of cardiac rhythm. When these many advances are ineffective, carefully selected patients can benefit from the support of mechanical hearts. Although these concepts were in the realm of science fiction in my student days, in future years as a cardiologist, I would be privileged to participate in and contribute to an outstanding period of advancement in medical care.

The last three years of medical study were in the major specialities: medicine, surgery and obstetrics. Medicine and surgery training was in the Richmond Hospital. Obstetrics and gynaecology training was in the Rotunda Lying-in Hospital, where a month of residence was required.[20] In this rather Rabelaisian den of heathen thought and behaviour, I learned not only about the physiological rudiments of pregnancy and birth but much about the whole business of existence. We were obliged to witness a specified number of births, the details of which had to be recorded and certified in a booklet by the sister in charge, who ruled as supreme as Hippolyta. Furthermore, she oversaw a function unique to the Rotunda: whereas all classical treatises on obstetrics agree that there are three stages of labour, the Rotunda devised a 'fourth stage', which demanded that having attended a delivery, students then washed the blood-drenched sheets in a sluice. This, we were told, was part of the ritual of conception, labour and birth. We complied without demur.

During the month in residence, we had to be available for 'district call' to the tenements in the neighbourhood where multiparous women were delivered at home rather than in hospital. These once majestic Georgian houses, which had housed the nobility in an earlier era, were now occupied by impoverished families. The occupants often accepted the misfortune of poverty with superlative dignity through the generosity and kindness they shared. The upper flats of these tenements were reached by wooden stairs on which the indentation of bygone footfalls had etched an undulating patina. I recall on one occasion as I trudged upwards to visit a woman who had given birth the night before, I met the father, a huge docker, who grunted to me as I made way for his enormous frame: 'By Jaysus, laddie, that was a right trap you set for me last night.' It took me some moments to absorb the brutal horror of this aside, in which he was alluding to the discomfort caused to him by small metal clips that had been used to suture his wife's vulva and vagina after an episiotomy to ease the delivery of her infant. I approached his wife's bedside overcome with grief for her, but she greeted me with a smile that dispelled any sympathetic sentiments as she proudly held out her newborn child for me to admire.

Students were paired for district deliveries, and it was customary to sit in Conway's Pub across from the hospital to await the call on a dedicated black phone. One such delivery remains etched in my mind. Clive, my Welsh student compatriot, and I departed for a nearby tenement. The father-to-be led us to where his wife lay in the throes of advanced labour. The room was cluttered with cooking items and cots temporarily emptied of offspring which had been transferred to the families in adjoining quarters. Despite her distress, this mother of many smiled a smile of smiles. She banished labour pain with a serenity of expression that broke across her ravished face like a tide of calmness after a tropical storm. With a gesture that was majestic – there's no other word for it – her left arm swept across the room encompassing the little that was hers and thereby bestowing it upon us. This moment of sensitivity was dispelled by the next contraction that brought tears to her eyes.

'Has the midwife arrived?' Clive asked, alarmed. The husband pointed to the water boiling on the stove and disappeared to the whispering corridors of the tenement as he had learned to do on previous occasions. The expectant mother reached for Clive's hand and guided his gloved fingers between her legs. Her cries shook the room. We laid drapes around her vagina that was widening with every cry as the black-haired head of the baby emerged. As the mother gave a sigh that seemed to sweep through the building, the head was through, and the rest of the little body gushed out in a flood of amnion and blood. For a terror-stricken moment of silence, we thought the infant was dead, but then we heard a gasp, followed by a cry as the baby entered its world of abject deprivation. The midwife arrived and dealt with the afterbirth. The infant lay between his mother's breasts. Her countenance radiated a beauty that even Piero della Francesca would have struggled to capture. The first cry of life was the signal for the tenement women to remove the soiled sheets and other paraphernalia. Then the proud father, and one or two close confrères, entered to admire his latest progeny. His face flushed with pride as he hauled a crate from under the bed. Everyone was offered a drink: the accoucheurs; the nurse; the women and men now crowding in from the tenement corridors, sensing a chance libation without the onus of recompense; and lastly, he served himself. 'A toast to the future – to the future of my son!' He raised his drink. Applause filled the room. Gazing proudly at her infant nuzzling blindly at her breasts, the mother reached for Clive's hand. 'Can I be so bold, Doctor,' she said with an alluring softness, 'to ask your name?' 'Of course,' he said, 'it's Jones.' 'I mean your first name.' 'Clive,' he said. 'I'm glad it's such a nice name,' she said, 'because that's what I am going to call my son.' A murmur of approval swept the gathering. Bottles were raised to the student whose handsome countenance was rendered all the more noble by tears welling up in his green Welsh eyes.

The final examinations in medicine, surgery and obstetrics were the culmination of six years of study. The exam had three parts. The first was an essay-format written exam. The second was the exacting 'clinical' exam where the student arrived at the appointed time at a designated hospital and was assigned to a patient. After taking a history and examining the patient, two consultants questioned the veracity of the history, asked the student to demonstrate the clinical abnormalities they found and then make a diagnosis. They would be questioned on the results of investigations, asked to propose the most appropriate treatment and give an opinion on the likely prognosis. The third part of the exam was a viva. The student sat at a table strewn with X-rays, ECG recordings, instruments and other items. Two consultants interrogated the student on aspects considered appropriate. In the case of a borderline student, they sought clarification on topics in which the examinee had shown a weakness. For a potential honours candidate, they would ask searching questions outside the expected repertoire of student knowledge. Based on this assessment process, the student was deemed suitable to be a 'doctor', or was destined to continue as a student for another period, after which the process would be repeated.

My final clinical obstetrics exam was in the Rotunda Hospital. I was assigned to a delightful woman, the mother of many children, who knew more about copulation, conception, pregnancy, delivery and life than was recorded in all the textbooks on these subjects. We warmed to each other immediately and she assured me that, having been the subject of so many examinations, she could help me tease out the intricacies of her obstetrical history and guide me to the abnormalities that made her worthy of being selected repeatedly for the exam. I accepted her guidance, and after I presented my findings to Professor Drew Davidson and an external examiner from Britain, they admitted that my presentation and conclusions were to their liking. The only problem arose when I realized that Davidson (whose drinking capacity was legendary, as was that of his co-examiner, a credential that no doubt earned his selection year after year) was about to allocate my marks to another candidate. I had to intervene to prevent this calamity. I returned later with a box of chocolates for my lovely mentor who had helped me towards undeserved honours. I don't remember my final medicine and surgical examinations with clarity, but I succeeded and was even awarded the hospital prizes.

After six years I now had to move from the relative ease of studentship to the responsibilities of being an actual doctor – a moment Ethna MacCarthy, doctor and poet, captured movingly in verse:

Ferreted from a five-year cave,
expelled from this earthy womb confused,
my eyes assaulted by the light,
I am at bay in feeble fear.[21]

In June 1963 I became a qualified doctor. The results of the final examination on the College noticeboard entitled me to introduce myself to all and sundry as 'Doctor O'Brien', an appellation not without significance in a society well used to doffing the cap to those with the titles of 'Father' or 'Doctor'. Of course, it would have been calamitous if I had failed the examinations, but my results, even with a smattering of honours in medicine and obstetrics, not so much saddened me but left me – and I cannot find a word precisely to describe my feeling – perhaps dispirited. A pivotal moment in my life had arrived, and nothing would ever be the same again. I walked away from the College, shunning the exhortations of my fellow students to join them in a celebratory drink. Instead, after phoning my mother to reassure her and my father that all was well, I walked across the road to St Stephen's Green and sat on a bench by the lake with a gaggle of ducks amusing themselves at my feet.

I sat there for an hour or more, pondering my newfound circumstances, trying to fathom why my mood was desultory rather than one of elation. I had been born into advantageous circumstances and was now privileged to be entering a career that offered me a prosperous future. The ducks quacked in agreement. A snowy-fleeced duck shat on my shoe. The omens are good, I thought as I raised myself from the bench to wipe my brogue in the grass.

Three tasks lay ahead before some celebratory imbibing. First, I went to a photo studio, as I promised my mother, to have this moment of achievement captured for posterity. The photograph was, and remains to this day, a sickening portrait of smug complacency. The second task, more pleasurable by far, was the selection of gold cufflinks for my father. The third task was, oddly, to 'buy' some cut-glass martini glasses with a decanter for my mother to store her beloved brew of gin and martini – all purchased by courtesy of the word 'doctor' that conveyed the illusion of prosperity to my creditors – a misapprehension that would lead to life-long indebtedness.

4. A Journey to Specialization

Let us emancipate the student, and give him time and opportunity for the cultivation of his mind, so that in his pupillage he shall not be a puppet in the hands of others, but rather a self-relying and reflecting being.
William Stokes, in Eoin O'Brien, *Conscience and Conflict: A Biography of Sir Dominic Corrigan, 1802–1880* (1983)

Within a week of qualifying, I became locum house physician at the City of Dublin Skin and Cancer Hospital for two weeks. Short though the period was, it's worth recounting it to indicate how times have changed. I slept in a room opposite a door to the basement bolted at night to keep the ghost of Andrew Charles (the founder of the hospital) confined. Indeed, strange sounds from the basement disturbed my sleep. Another interruption was a nurse's inevitable knock on the door to fetch morphine for a patient in distress. I was the custodian of dangerous drugs, locked in a safe and released only after many forms had been signed and countersigned. My medical duties were not onerous: a ward round with Matron in the morning, an occasional call to ease the suffering of a patient with terminal cancer and, sadly, the issuing of death certificates. Breakfast was served in bed! When I suggested to the porter that this was an excessive luxury, he dismissed it with a phrase that still resonates: 'But Jaysus, Doctor, the man before you refused to budge from his bed until I had brought him his lunch!'

Although I was permitted to use the title 'doctor', I was not allowed to practise medicine until I had completed a one-year internship in my teaching hospital, the Richmond. I was house physician to Professor Alan Thompson for the first six months,[1] and for my surgical internship I was attached to Paddy Carey, a hardworking neurosurgeon, whom I came to respect greatly. I called him in the small hours of many nights to deal with neurosurgical emergencies. He never demurred, and I often assisted him in theatre, followed by breakfast in the 'crow's nest' – a kitchen haven high above the operating theatres.[2]

Research wasn't a predominant activity in the Richmond, with two notable exceptions. The first was Alan Mooney, the ophthalmologist, who working quietly and diligently, published his careful observations. I welcomed our discussions on the eye as a window to neurological illnesses. The second was the former head of neurosurgery, Adams McConnell, who had an international reputation and was regarded in Dublin as the pioneer of the speciality of neurosurgery. I was surprised one day to see McConnell walking the wards accompanied only by a loyal sister; being retired, he was no longer accompanied by the usual entourage of doctors and nurses. To ameliorate this indignity, I escaped from other duties to accompany him and was rewarded by the wisdom of his vast experience, which often led to a diagnosis in patients with perplexing symptoms. His opinion, written with a pencil stub in the hospital notes, was invariably a gem of intuition. McConnell also taught me that brevity could be the essence of expression.[3]

I became adept at performing lumbar puncture to diagnose subarachnoid haemorrhage and suspected meningitis. I performed air encephalograms, a procedure in which spinal fluid is replaced with air to outline the cavities in the brain. I assisted in the tedious procedure of stereotaxis for Parkinson's disease, which involved ablating areas of the brain with an electrode introduced through a hole drilled in the skull. The procedure's success was gauged by the patient's assessment of whether the disease's characteristic tremor had abated – this was before controlled clinical trials became mandatory, and success was based on anecdotal rather than scientific fact.[4]

I also assisted the neuro-anaesthetists. Johnny Conroy, a music-loving raconteur who could recount in vivid detail the latest Wagnerian renditions from his annual visit to the Bayreuth Festival, was a close friend, but I had most contact with Paul Murray, a touchy former rugby international, whose tetchiness I had to confront on more than one occasion.[5] He prepared patients for hypothermia, and

I fetched the buckets of ice needed to cool patients so that the oxygen requirement of the cerebral cells was reduced before brain surgery.

I encountered many tragedies in the Richmond, which was then the national centre for neurosurgery: patients maimed in motor accidents; debilitated by strokes; convulsing because of brain cancer; in delirium from meningitis – all were transferred to the Richmond. I have a sad memory of a young Englishman on a business trip to Dublin. On the way from the airport in a taxi, the car door swung open and he fell out, striking his head on a kerb. He was rushed to the neurosurgical department, where, despite efforts to evacuate a brain haemorrhage, he died. The next day Geraghty, the urbane head porter who manned the foyer, sought me out in a state of grave concern to tell me the deceased's fiancée had arrived and wished to discuss his progress. He ushered her to the staff room so that the news could be broken to her in quietude, but as all the senior staff were in theatre, I had to face the responsibility. This beautiful young woman broke down in disbelief and cried on my shoulder. They were to be married in a month. She was alone in Dublin. All I could do was arrange for someone who knew her fiancé to collect her and look after her. The pain of this encounter and my self-perceived clumsiness in offering support endures to this day.

During my internship I made many friends: Dermot Byrnes, Joseph Mary Kelly, Frank Hogan, Mariana Goulandris, Nuala McLean and Celia Fiennes, the mention of whom brings an amusing incident to mind. Celia and I were tasked to organize the annual hospital dance in the Gresham Hotel. After visiting the hotel to make final arrangements, we sped back to the hospital on Celia's scooter. As we flew past the Four Courts, a huge policeman raised a mighty hand and brought us to a halt. He even placed his boot against the front wheel lest we tried to make a run for it. I decided to do the talking since I feared that Celia's English accent might not bode well for us. In response to his query as to where we thought we were speeding to, I explained we were doctors returning from a mission of mercy en route to the Richmond Hospital. Unimpressed, he took out a grubby notebook and the butt of a pencil from a cavernous pocket. Licking the pencil, he boomed: 'What's youse names?' I informed him that the driver was Dr Celia Twisleton-Wykeham-Fiennes. Drawing a deep breath through his cyanosed lips, he closed his notebook and warned: 'If I ever see youse pair speeding round this corner on that yoke without regard for the life of all and sundry, I will clamp youse both in jail.'

My first post after my internship was as a paediatric house officer in the Rotunda, where I was known simply as the 'Baby Doctor'. I was attached to two paediatricians, Professor Eric Doyle and Dr Patrick McClancy. One of my duties was to sit with McClancy performing exchange transfusions in babies with jaundice, making polite conversation for hours as I recorded the quantity of exchanged blood. My major role, however, was to tour the city in a van emblazoned with INFANT SERVICE – ROTUNDA HOSPITAL. Having delivered a premature infant in a tenement building, a midwife would request the Baby Doctor. Donned in a white coat, I'd set off in the van, siren blazing. Occasionally a roaming garda car assisted me to my destination. On arrival, I would run up the tenement stairs with warm blankets and assure the mother that her infant (now in my arms) would be back in a few days. Then I'd descend from this well of poverty with my firmly wrapped charge, which I would place gently in the incubator in the back of the van. Then off at full speed to the Rotunda, where I'd wheel the incubator with its precious cargo to the infant care unit. A remarkable sister, Maudie Moran, would transfer the baby to a more elaborate incubator. We would then enjoy tea, discussing the progress of my previous cargo, now thriving in the warmth and security of an adjoining incubator. Maudie taught me all I would ever need to know about infant prematurity and life itself. I have very dear memories of her.

I was joined in the Rotunda by the Gingerman of medicine, Eugene O'Connor, who, with his lust for life and fun, soon became a close friend. Eugene studied medicine at University College Galway, where he found life so convivial, he spent well over the years prescribed to learn the art of medicine. The denizens of the city interpreted this phenomenon not as a failure but as the college's obligation not to let him leave 'until he knew everything'.[6]

And then there was the moustachioed Paddy O'Grady, corpulent *bon vivant* with no moral scruples other than to dote on his much-loved widowed mother with her collection of Beule furniture. With a laugh to dispel the gloomiest thoughts on the darkest of days, he was given to utterances of invective against Catholicism – and where more appropriately than within the hallowed walls of that Protestant bastion of midwifery, the Rotunda.

I moved from the Rotunda to Cherry Orchard Fever Hospital in Ballyfermot,[7] which lives on in memory for good reason. Two infective illnesses, which were prevalent, had to be diagnosed accurately – streptococcal throat had to be distinguished from diphtheria, and chickenpox had to be differentiated from the remote but ever-present threat of smallpox. Here I realized how the thermometer – a simple clinical device – could be the harbinger of mischief. Patients with poliomyelitis occupied one of the ward blocks. Whereas the virus usually affected the spinal or peripheral nerves, in these unfortunate patients, the nerves transmitting the impulses for the respiratory muscles were affected, causing paralysis of breathing and death if the patient didn't receive artificial respiratory support. One such measure was the iron lung, a negative pressure ventilator, which took over the breathing function with a regular pumping rhythm to provide mechanical inflation and deflation of the paralysed respiratory muscles. However, the price of survival was confinement in an encircling chamber, which one patient described as lying in a coffin with one's head sticking out.[8]

Daily, I faced the horrific fate of young patients confined to the iron lung. It made me feel so unwell there were times I couldn't face doing a round in the building in which they were housed. I would phone the sister, saying I had a cold and feared infecting the patients. But mostly, I persevered. I would sit at the head of one of these frightening devices, chatting to the encased and stoical victim fated to live inside it. The selfish rumination *There but for the grace of God go I* ran in my mind. As a child I had been sent to the Gaeltacht to learn Irish but shortly after I arrived, a polio epidemic broke out and I was sent home – thankfully, I avoided the virus.

Cherry Orchard Fever Hospital influenced my future in another profound way. One morning my fellow house officer, Jim O'Connell, and I were having coffee when he was phoned by a friend, Tona, to whom he apologized for not being able to accompany her to a party that evening as he was on duty. He handed the phone to me, suggesting I should go instead. He thereby introduced me to the woman who would become my wife and the most enduring influence in my life.

In searching for future directions, I looked in desperation to America. Peter McLean, a resident in surgery at the Mayo Clinic in Rochester, Minnesota (who would later achieve distinction for performing the first kidney transplant in Ireland), invited me to apply for a fellowship in the Mayo. The interview involved being assessed by department heads and other staff and being taken to lunch, the purpose of which (I sensed) was to see if I could hold a knife and fork and conduct a conversation. The visit ended pleasantly over dinner with Peter and his wife, Nuala, whom I knew from the Richmond where she had been an intern when I was a student. I was offered a four-year fellowship in haematology. Why haematology? I can't remember, but I declined. I saw a fellowship at the Mayo akin to entering a seminary where nothing would be wanting, but the stipend would be so meagre that even an escape to the Twin Cities – the only cultural outlet within reach – would be impossible. I next considered Baltimore. I was offered a job in what was then known as the Baltimore General Hospital, but the

Vietnam War decided me against it. Having an abhorrence of violence, I wasn't prepared to be drafted to fight for a country endeavouring to impose democracy in a Buddhist country in distant Southeast Asia. And so, with Gerry Herlihy, a fellow doctor and his wife, who were also planning to go to the US, we decided against doing so and tore up our contracts in Neary's, tipping a pint to the US and to any gods that might give guidance to two jobless doctors.

Those gods threw me into the company of Dr Patrick J. Rafferty. He was a year or two ahead of me in medical college and had just been appointed to a large general practice in Birmingham, or to be more precise Smethwick – one of the most deprived suburbs of that sprawling metropolis. He was searching for a junior partner and persuaded me to fill this role.

I spent over a year in general practice in Smethwick, where I coped with illnesses in a mixed population prone to diseases determined by genetic and racial peculiarities and poverty. The poverty in this maelstrom of ethnicity was far removed from Dublin, where the black and brown demographic was composed almost exclusively of medical students. In Smethwick, political debate was put into perspective with the slogan daubed by a graffitist on the outer wall of our surgery: 'If you want a nigger for a neighbour, vote Labour'.

There were three surgeries, one of which was a dark, rat-infested shack on Queen Street, which we demolished when the practice was later amalgamated into one surgery. In my experience, which had been hospital-based, general practitioners (GPs) were considered inferior to consultants. In Smethwick, I quickly revised this mistakenly elitist view. Here, GPs were the backbone of the health service. I developed a high regard for the National Health Service (NHS), which Aneurin Bevan introduced in 1948, despite the opposition of the doctors in the British Medical Association (BMA), whose mouths 'he stuffed with gold'. The NHS was the first truly universal health care system, and it remains a remarkable monument, outliving many ill-advised adjustments by politicians, who have failed to appreciate its fundamental value and importance to the health of the British nation.

Under the NHS, one of the provisions on offer to GPs altered the course of my future. To minimize hospital referrals to out-patient departments, GPs could request a hospital consultant to see patients in their surgeries, and the consultant would be duly reimbursed. I used this service to engage Dr Alex Paton, a gastroenterologist with a special interest in liver disease in Dudley Road Hospital, to see patients about whom I needed expert advice.

During one of these consultations, Paton, who discerned uncertainty in my desire to be a GP, invited me to attend his teaching class in Dudley Road, which he gave once a week for doctors preparing for the membership exam of the Royal College of Physicians in London. I joined ten or so doctors attending his membership rounds, which were masterful exercises in clinical teaching delivered with humour and enthusiasm, often laced with the thrust of wit and sarcasm. On one occasion, he turned to me with the upheld wrist of a Wiltshire farmer on which there was a nasty-looking skin lesion: 'O'Brien, here we have a classic example of Orf – take a close look and describe the features and then give us a learned dissertation on Orf.' I took the wrist and gave a dermatological description of the sore, but never having heard of Orf, I could only declare that it was 'a truly orful disease'. Paton made me realize that my future lay in hospital medicine. Later, after I returned to Dublin to pursue that future, he would re-enter my life and greatly influence my destiny.

General practice humbled me. Here I was in a country among people who differed from me, and I from them, in so many ways that we viewed one another with curiosity and a need to comprehend the origins of such diversity. How was it that, despite the similarities of colour, physiognomy, language and geographical proximity, the Irish could be so different from the English? Of course, there was the animosity of centuries, which could be dragged from history to explain it, but there were moments when the British sense of superiority, spawned perhaps by the colonial ethos that remained undiminished for some, emerged to denigrate discussion. When unleashed, this spirit of self-righteousness instilled insensitivity into humour and could be hurtful. But there were discerning people too, who respected our differences. For example, in rugby sallies and medical meetings to Scotland and Wales, a common Celtic bond created a warmer relationship. In England in the 1960s, Anglo–Irish relationships were strained and destined to deteriorate substantially in the next decade but I was offered the hand of friendship, based on my individuality rather than my origins.

In England it became necessary to share the comparatively liberal mores to which I was now exposed. Coming from a land where contraception was banned and sexual union was countenanced only for procreation, I had to come to terms with abortion, a word that was murmured in hushed tones by liberal thinkers in the Free State. In Smethwick, many women regarded abortion as an inalienable right. I had to reconcile whatever principles of morality arose from a religious indoctrination with the reality of practising medicine among an impoverished populace with no moral disagreement with abortion. I decided to contradict Catholicism on this issue.

I also had to confront a tender issue for doctors: palliative care. In the 1960s a general practitioner carried potent drugs, including heroin. As a result, it was possible, without invoking the concept of euthanasia, to ease the pain of terminal illness. I recall a patient who lived in a particularly poor quarter of Smethwick. The family consisted of the dying father, his wife, two daughters and a son. I gave him the sad news that he had only weeks to live. He asked that the family hear the prognosis. All pledged their support so that he would die at home, and I would do what I could to ease his suffering. I visited often to chat with the father whose innate philosophy appealed to me. As his illness advanced rapidly, so too did his suffering. The family cared for him with great tenderness, taking turns to nurse him during the night when spectres haunted his troubled dreams. On one of my morning visits, he called for his wife and children. When all were gathered, he told me they all decided he should have no more pain. He had no god to make peace with – neither he nor his family believed in the hereafter. The dying man held my hand in gratitude, and his tearful wife embraced me. Later, I watched the father sleep in his wife's embrace, his son and daughters around his bed. He slept peacefully into death, and I left the family to comfort themselves after his gentle passing. General practice taught me much about life – and death.

After a year in general practice, I returned to Dublin and to hospital medicine. I was appointed as medical registrar to Professor Mervyn Abrahamson and was awarded a research fellowship in the Fibrinolytic Laboratory in the Richmond Hospital and in the Houston Cancer Research laboratory in the College of Surgeons under the directorship of Professor Alan Thompson and Dr R. Douglas Thornes. My initiation in research was unusual. Thornes's background in scientific research was haphazard; his hospital attachments were ephemeral and dependent on financial support from the pharmaceutical industry.[9] During an appointment to Johns Hopkins University, he collaborated with another scientist, Professor Sumner Wood Jr, who developed the technique of time-lapse photography to demonstrate that warfarin could inhibit the locomotion of cancer cells without affecting normal cells. Thornes extended this line of research to show that cancer cells, once deprived of a protective fibrin hideaway, could be reached by effective drugs. I met Sumner Wood when he visited Dublin, and his sudden death by suicide at the early age of forty-four in 1974 was a great loss to science, and indeed to Dublin, where his scientific expertise was beginning to influence promising collaborative research.

Thornes abhorred committing research to paper. Since I enjoyed writing, he left it to me to prepare our work for publication. From 1968 to 1969, we published five papers. Looking critically at these now, all but one lacked finesse. This paper was published in *The Lancet*, and it earned encouraging editorial comment.[10] The most frustrating reflection of this period of research is my lack of serendipitous flair that should have led me to recognize that the fibrinolytic enzyme protease, which we were studying in cancer research, had far greater potential to dissolve clots in arteries, and was one of the first so-called 'clot-busting drugs' that are now commonplace in the treatment of heart attack and stroke.

Tona and I, who had been living together for some time, decided to marry and, not yet having abandoned religion altogether, we favoured an evening wedding to avoid the tedium that often characterized morning weddings and ended in Bacchus-induced rancour. However, the Catholic Church refused to marry us in the evening, until we threatened the church with the alternative of civil marriage. A compromise was agreed – we could have an evening ceremony without the customary mass. We were married in University Church on the evening of 27 May 1968, with Pat Rafferty as best man and Maura Lee as bridesmaid. This was followed by a reception in the RCSI and later by less formal wining and dining with friends in the Old Cod restaurant on Lincoln Place. As night progressed to dawn, the more gregarious trooped back to our flat on St Stephen's Green to conclude the celebrations.

By now I was five years qualified and going nowhere – it was time to take stock. Perusing the 'positions vacant' pages of the medical journals, I saw that Dr Alex Paton was advertising for a general medicine and gastroenterology registrar at Dudley Road Hospital in Birmingham. I applied despite my shortcomings. I would be competing against candidates with academic backgrounds, whereas I carried the incubus of holding a licentiate from the RCSI rather than a degree from a university. In addition, I would be an Irish applicant among many British doctors. Moreover, a year in general practice wasn't advantageous for specialist training. However, despite these weaknesses, I was shortlisted and went to Birmingham to be interviewed by four consultants, one of whom was Paton.

I defended my year in general practice by expanding on the lessons I'd learned about the difficulties of my patients' lives in an impoverished environment.

I stated that I had no regrets about having worked on the NHS's front line of medical care. Having let his colleagues expose my many weaknesses, Paton asked me to give an account of the work I had published in *The Lancet*. I expounded on the relatively unknown fibrinolytic system on which I was well versed, having read the monograph by the acknowledged world authority, George Fearnley, in Gloucestershire Royal Hospital, whom I had also visited to discuss my research. However, the kernel of Paton's curiosity was to ascertain who had written *The Lancet* article. I explained that because Thornes preferred laboratory experimentation to writing, I assembled the piece. This won me the job.

In October 1968 I took up duty at Dudley Road Hospital, an institution that would greatly influence my understanding of medicine and my approach to illness.[11] My first night as Resident Medical Officer is as clear today as if it happened yesterday. I introduced myself to the telephonist from whom I collected my bleep. In sending me on my way, he nonchalantly informed me that the catchment area was 3.5 million people, a statistic that put my new job into a daunting perspective; it equated with being on call for the entire island of Ireland, a realistic assessment, as I would soon learn. Being a gastroenterologist with expertise in liver disease, many patients were referred to Paton for treatment of alcoholic liver disease, which was rife in Birmingham and I became experienced in its management. Although my main allegiance was to Paton, I worked with other consultants, admitting their patients and assisting at their out-patient sessions.[12]

Patients with every kind of illness flooded through the doors of casualty every day, providing me with experience that would later stand me in good stead. Apart from treating illnesses with which I was familiar (diabetic coma, severe asthma, strokes, kidney failure, heart attack and meningitis), I was now treating patients from India and Pakistan with advanced tuberculosis, trying to lower blood pressure in young patients with malignant hypertension, coping with patients vomiting blood from oesophageal varices owing to alcoholic liver failure and treating patients with sickle cell disease, a genetic illness which was then virtually unknown in Dublin.

I had to identify the personal turmoil that motivated a suicidal gesture as distinct from a genuine intention to end life. One memory still disturbs me. A young man aged thirty had taken a large quantity of a sleeping tablet, Mandrax. Apart from coma and circulatory depression, he developed the life-threatening complication of pulmonary oedema from fluid flooding the lungs. I spent the night washing out the excess fluid with intravenous diuretics while correcting the fall in his blood pressure and heart rate. When he regained consciousness, I was sitting by his bedside, and with a certain complacency, if not pride, that we had saved him, I told him he would be all right. Disbelief crossed his handsome face: 'Christ, you're not telling me I'm still alive?' I learned how the breakdown of his homosexual relationship and his ostracization from family and society had culminated in his suicide attempt. When leaving the hospital days later, he thanked me, adding with a wry smile that he would make sure I was not on duty when he made his next attempt. We shook hands, each knowing that the crossing of our paths would have lasting effects on us both.

In the late 1960s a hospital phenomenon existed that has now passed into history – the 'hospital mess'. The mess housed interns and senior house officers (mostly unmarried) in modest rooms for six months. In addition, there were rooms for registrars, like me, who lived outside the hospital but were required to live-in while on duty. The mess was a place of vibrant conviviality brought about by the mingling of personnel sharing common and demanding duties. Here doctors from the three major disciplines of medicine, surgery and obstetrics discussed the difficulties peculiar to each other's speciality. Meals were served in a large dining room. A TV room doubled as a reading space. However, most popular was the bar, where each doctor had a tab that was payable monthly. The bar was under the stewardship of the mess president, who appointed a treasurer to oversee its management. I was duly elected mess president. One of my tasks was to obtain sponsorship from pharmaceutical companies to support a monthly shindig attended by the consultant staff (usually without spouses), the resident doctors, the nurses and paramedical staff, such as radiographers and technicians. The highlight of the social calendar was the Christmas party when the staff presented 'life in a hospital' with satirical and risqué vignettes.

Joan Patey, the sister in charge of Paton's male-patients ward, was remarkable. She carried in her mind not only the medical and therapeutic details of each patient but their social and family circumstances that would determine the home support needed after their discharge. She knew the idiosyncrasies of each team member and often tipped me off to the personal stresses of junior doctors. She was also prepared to confront senior staff if she believed they were acting unreasonably.

One morning, after a busy night during which I had treated a patient in a diabetic coma in whom maintaining potassium levels had been a challenge, I was pleased to present a lucid and conversing patient to Paton. However, being in one of his irascible moods, Paton, using derisory language, criticized my management of the patient because the latest potassium level had dipped in response to his large insulin requirement. This was a welcome diversion for the team, who enjoyed a little drama to enliven the ward round. Paton gave me no opportunity to respond, and, realizing that I had to make a stand if I was to retain the team's respect, I beckoned him out of earshot. I advised him quietly that if he wanted me to continue on rounds, he had to apologize. What I didn't know until later was that Patey had marched Paton to her office, where she told him his behaviour was reprehensible. He apologized, acknowledging that he had reacted in the patient's best interests. I admitted that tiredness made me behave petulantly. We returned to the team discussing the latest approach to managing low insulin levels with a new and promising drug called glucagon, and Paton asked me to give the team a brief account of its place in managing diabetes. We never crossed swords again.

Paton was one of the most delightfully eccentric personalities I encountered in medicine. He was sceptical of administrative processes, often preferring to bypass the Medical Board to avoid wasting time and inviting troublesome interference from indecisive colleagues. His irascibility could be both exasperating and amusing. His colleagues believed his behaviour made him 'fucking impossible', but such appraisals often overlooked his many unique and endearing qualities.[13]

The relentless imperative of studying for the membership exam to one of the Royal Colleges, without which a junior doctor could not proceed to consultant status, added to the stress of being frequently on hospital duty. The exams were formidable: one rarely passed on the first attempt – a misfortune for candidates but a substantial source of income for the Colleges. I attended Maurice Pappworth's membership course in London on Paton's recommendation. Pappworth had remarkable success in coaching generations of doctors from around the world. When asked to what he attributed his successful reputation, he replied: 'I just teach them tricks.' Coming from Dublin, where I had enjoyed the wit and thrust of Jewish humour, I appreciated Pappworth's sense of fun, and we became friends. 'Statistics', he said, 'are like bikinis, concealing what is vital, whilst revealing much that is occasionally interesting.' His invective was often directed at establishment figures whose ranks he was, ironically, enhancing with his course.

In 1969 I also attended a course in advanced medicine at the Hammersmith Hospital in London, where I learned a great deal from three eminent cardiologists, John Goodwin, Celia Oakley and John Shillingford. All were international figures and influential in my selecting cardiology as a future speciality. I was present in the Hammersmith for the first clinical presentation of an echocardiogram, a technique that would dramatically advance diagnostic cardiology.

In March 1971 I put myself forward for the Royal College of Physicians of Ireland membership. The exam began with a three-hour essay paper in the Corrigan Hall of the College, followed by a clinical exam in Sir Patrick Dun's Hospital. Hospitals kept a list of patients who had 'classical signs' of a disease and could give a good account of their complaints. I was taken to my first 'major case'. As I approached the bedside, I diagnosed the female patient's illness simply because she had the classical facial discoloration known as the 'mitral facies', in which the skin of the nose and cheeks develop a purplish colour in patients with long-standing rheumatic disease of the mitral valve. I knew her pulse would be irregular because of atrial fibrillation, which invariably develops in such patients. I surmised she might have some degree of heart failure, but that diuretic treatment would have been given to control this, especially if she had come into hospital solely for the exam rather than being an in-patient. What I did not know was how many valves of her heart might be affected by the rheumatic illness.

In a clinical exam, one of the first tasks is to win over the patient rather than let any brusqueness be a cause of disharmony. My patient was a delightful lady who, having participated in numerous membership exams, was experienced in putting the examinee at ease. We warmed to each other immediately. Her history was classical for rheumatic cardiac disease. I showed that she had advanced disease of the cardiac valves with multiple cardiac murmurs audible with the stethoscope. She also had the clinical signs of treated cardiac failure. One of my examiners, a general physician, was the one I needed to impress most. The other examiner was an endocrinologist who, not being an authority on cardiac diagnoses, I feared might wish to impress his co-examiner by inferring that my appraisal was inaccurate. I presented the history, the symptoms and the clinical abnormalities with a summary of the diagnoses. The endocrinologist asked me to explain the cause of the mitral facies. I was questioned on my findings and had to defend my diagnosis of aortic regurgitation, which neither seemed convinced was present, but when I demonstrated the classical clinical manifestations, they agreed with the diagnosis. Next was a discussion as to how I would manage the patient and if I would recommend further surgery. Apparently satisfied, the examiners took me to the 'minor cases' where I was shown a patient with severe rheumatoid arthritis of the hand, another with changes of diabetes in the retina when I examined his eyes with an ophthalmoscope, another with a peripheral neuropathy of the hands, another with acromegaly and finally a patient with classical Parkinson's disease.

The following day I was called for a viva. The examiners were two physicians in possession of the comments from my essay paper and the clinical exam.

The session started with pleasantries about how I viewed British compared to Irish medicine. I was careful to extol the standard in the homeland while observing that the main difference in Britain was exposure to diseases such as sickle cell anaemia, which was unknown in Ireland. As I had hoped, this led to my being questioned on the illness. An ECG showing heart block led to a discussion on temporary pacing, which I performed regularly in Dudley Road Hospital, and the examination ended positively.

The following day I received the news that I'd passed the exam. Relieved, I went to the Toby Jug and downed a pint of Guinness. Frank Swift – the owner who had seen me through many moments of financial insecurity during my six-year medical apprenticeship by advancing me drink against the surety of a well-worn Omega watch that once belonged to my father – greeted me as a long-lost friend. I told Frank I had passed the exam, and, knowing it was a significant milestone, he paid me the highest honour his establishment could bestow by inviting me to join him for lunch in his living quarters during the so-called 'holy hour' when the pub had to close. We ascended the rickety stairs to a kitchen with a large sink into which Swift urinated and in which he then proceeded to peel some potatoes, which he threw into a saucepan with some cabbage. From a large fridge came ham, which he carved while recounting tales of bygone patrons of the Toby Jug. I listened enraptured, enjoying another pint of Guinness. Such moments are rare. Frank (whom I would be destined to care for later when he developed cirrhosis of the liver) and the Toby Jug are no more, but the occasion lives on in my fondness for paradoxes because surely this was one of the strangest. Here I was, freshly admitted to the Royal College of Physicians of Ireland while simultaneously being admitted to the inner sanctum of Swift's eccentric emporium of life and booze.

Returning to Birmingham, I told Paton I had passed my Irish membership. He shrugged and said, 'When are you sitting the London membership?' then returned to reading the *British Medical Journal*. A month later, I sat the membership exam of the Royal College of Physicians of London, the premier membership exam at that time.[14] Although I recall little of the event, I did write an appreciative piece in the *British Medical Journal* acknowledging the kindness of the sister in St Bartholomew's Hospital in London who had welcomed me with strawberries and cream. Not surprisingly she, rather than the examiners, lives on in my memory[15] – another of life's paradoxes. Upon returning to Dudley Road, I entered Paton's office, less ebulliently this time, casually informing him of my success in London. This news brought a very different response to the earlier mention of my success in the Irish membership exam; he stood up and, putting his arm around my shoulder, said, 'Now we're talking!'

It was time to decide to which speciality I would devote my professional life. Paton wanted me to continue in gastroenterology, but I was fascinated by cardiology. So, difficult though it was to part company with Paton, I moved to cardiology.

I was fortunate to be trained by John Mackinnon, the head of a small Department of Cardiology at Dudley Road. He was the finest clinical cardiologist I would ever have the privilege of knowing. He was considerate with patients, and his skill with the stethoscope was sublime. He was a gentleman in the true sense of that word, who placed the patient at the centre of all clinical deliberation. He trained me not only in clinical cardiology but also in cardiac catheterisation, where his interpretation of information was cautious and his approach to investigation and intervention was conservative rather than aggressive.[16]

Innovations in science and technology would have had little impact on cardiological practice were it not for the establishment of coronary care units (CCUs) throughout the world in the 1960s.[17] The CCU in Dudley Road was a cordoned-off section of a general ward. Here, new concepts were tried and tested to reduce the unacceptable mortality rate of 40 per cent in patients suffering from a heart attack. The introduction of a novel technique known as cardiopulmonary resuscitation (CPR) gave doctors the means to revive patients after a heart attack, whereas previously such patients would be pronounced dead. Cessation of cardiac activity was accepted as irreversible and inviolate and attempts to interfere with what was regarded as an almost divine inevitability were relegated to the realms of Frankensteinian fiction. After the 1960s it was shown that adequate circulation could be maintained during cardiac arrest by external chest compression.[18] With this dramatic advance, CPR became applicable at any place or time and could be performed by trained lay people without a medical background. The process of bringing the 'briefly dead' back to life needed just one other technological advance, which came with a device known as a defibrillator that could administer a direct current shock to paralyze the fibrillating ventricles and allow the natural pacemaker to retake control by restoring regular normal rhythm. In 1966 Frank Pantridge at the Royal Victoria Hospital in Belfast introduced the first mobile defibrillator unit and implemented the concept of mobile coronary care. As a result, he is known as 'the father of emergency medicine'. He created the era of heart-attack management outside the hospital. The need for lightweight, battery-operated defibrillators became obvious, and subsequent research focused on reducing the size of these life-saving devices.[19]

The CPR routine in Dudley Road was typical of CPR practice across the UK in the 1960s. The process was initiated by the 999 bleep, signalling to those on the resuscitation rota to rush to the scene of the cardiac arrest. A designated nurse brought a resuscitation trolley with all the necessary drugs, a defibrillator, endotracheal tubes and oxygen. The first medic on the scene moved the patient to the floor and commenced mouth-to-mouth respiration and cardio-pulmonary massage until the anaesthetist arrived and intubated the patient while another doctor continued intermittent rhythmic massage of the chest wall to maintain circulation. The drill was well-planned and well-rehearsed. One nurse logged the events, and the anaesthetist inserted an endotracheal tube to ensure ventilation with oxygen and cannulas were inserted to provide access to the circulatory system. The CCU nurse ensured that the electrodes attached to the patient gave a clear and uninterrupted electrocardiographic record of the patient's cardiac rhythm.

My role was to direct CPR proceedings. I gave instruction for each successive phase of operation. After each intervention, after every drug administration, intravenously, or as each failed action demanded more extreme measures (such as the injection of adrenaline directly into the heart) all eyes were drawn to the monitor to see if the fibrillary waves of ventricular fibrillation had been converted to normal sinus rhythm. A brief flicker of ventricular fibrillation was the cue for me to take control of the shock electrodes and deliver direct current shocks while ensuring the team were not in danger of themselves being shocked. Again, all eyes would watch the screen. The 999 team continued like this, however despondent or drained they might be, until I gave the order to stop. This was always a difficult decision. But the team were at one in that once the decision was made, it was final.

A failed resuscitation, however, was the beginning of another process: the onerous tidying up of the intimate immediacies of a life just departed. Each team member recorded the events, the drugs given, the shocks administered, the responses to each intervention and, depressingly, the ultimate outcome. The sister-in-charge oversaw removal of the intravenous lines, the urinary catheter and the cleaning of the bloodied evidence of intervention at the access sites to the circulatory system – the neck, the groin, the antecubital fossa. Scorch marks to the chest were effaced, and then the lifeless body of the patient was placed on clean sheets in preparation for the family to see their beloved without a hint of the dramatic turmoil that was the prelude to what might be regarded as an undignified departure. But was it undignified? Certainly, at first glance there is little dignity to the picture of four or five people in white coats and nursing uniforms clamouring over a defenceless being and invading, with their relentless catheters, tubes, drugs and electricity, the innermost organs of life. A sense of despair and futility was inevitable after an unsuccessful resuscitation, but we had to balance the despondency of failure with the act of daring to fail in the first place. The many instances of success offset the hopelessness of loss.

I learnt many lessons as the resuscitation movement progressed, not only in managing acute medical catastrophes but also in the philosophy of existence – the meaning of life. For example, a patient I called 'the dollmaker' was admitted to the CCU with a heart attack. He went into ventricular fibrillation, and the resuscitation team was called. The initial shock brought him back to normal sinus rhythm, which lasted only minutes before further shocks were required. The acidosis caused by the cessation of cardiac function was corrected by an infusion of bicarbonate, and his potassium level was corrected. But the heart rhythm continued to revert to the flickering, ineffective contractions of ventricular fibrillation. After twenty shocks the team were exhausted, but the circulation had been maintained and I instructed them to continue with resuscitation. Eventually, after thirty shocks, the cardiac rhythm stabilized, and the dollmaker recovered consciousness.

During the night, I checked on his progress. He knew how close to the 'other side' he had been and assured me that the experience wasn't unpleasant, but I knew how perilously close he still was to crossing that divide. Later his heart rate slowed to thirty beats per minute owing to the development of heart block. This indicated damage to the delicate conducting system on which the heart depended for the transmission of electrical impulses from the heart's pacemaker to the ventricles. It was a particularly ominous complication in a patient with a heart attack. We wheeled him to the radiology department where, under X-ray control, I passed a temporary pacing wire through a vein in his arm to the apex of his left ventricle and then set the pacemaker to pass an electrical impulse to the ventricle so that it would contract regularly, seventy times per minute, and prevent the body, and especially the brain, from being deprived of oxygen. Over the next week, the dollmaker's condition stabilized. I remember the first day he walked flanked by the sister and nurse, whose prettiness he commented on with an approving wink.

His first visit in out-patients still kindles a sense of poignant affection. The day was cold and wet. As I helped him to take off his soaked coat, I commented on what a bloody awful day it was. He took my hand and, looking me in the eye, said in words that derived from the experience of having sensed the closeness of death: 'No, Dr O'Brien, every day is a good day.' He rummaged in a bag and brought out a doll he had made as a gift of gratitude for giving him a new lease of life. This beautiful doll, with every detail of the famous Rupert Bear, painstakingly reproduced, remains with me to the present day and is a constant reminder of the ephemerality of existence.

As CPR improved, so too did the success rate. However, in the 1960s it was often applied indiscriminately in the misguided belief that resuscitation was possible in all circumstances. Patients with fatal illnesses, many of whom were elderly, were subjected to CPR. Some doctors saw CPR as an opportunity to issue a personal vendetta to the prince of death. This was before the do-not-resuscitate (DNR) order was formulated into an ethical policy.

Constant monitoring of patients in a CCU after a heart attack not only allowed detection of the fast heart rate of ventricular fibrillation as a potentially fatal occurrence, but slowing of the heart, which might also be calamitous, could be identified. CCUs now began to provide the technique of temporary pacing to such patients whereby an electrode could be passed into a vein in the groin or arm to the right ventricle, where it could be wedged under radiographic control and then attached to a battery-powered pacemaker that would stimulate the ventricles to contract at a normal rate of sixty to seventy beats per minute. After some days the patient's wounded heart recovered sufficiently to initiate the normal rhythm of the heart and the temporary pacemaker could be removed. I inserted hundreds of temporary pacemakers during my time as cardiac registrar in Dudley Road Hospital.

Apart from the need for pacing in the stunned heart after a heart attack, there was another indication for the newly developed methodology of artificial pacing, which could also be managed in the CCU. In some people the specialized pacing tissue in the heart degenerates with age so that the heart slows and is unable to provide oxygenated blood to the brain and if the heart beats very slowly, consciousness is lost. This condition, first described by two Irish doctors – one a surgeon, Robert Adams, and the other a physician, William Stokes (the same Stokes who propagated the use of the stethoscope) - is known to this day as a 'Stokes-Adams attack'.[20]

As cardiac registrar, it was my responsibility to perform temporary pacing and then liaise with the surgeon for insertion of a permanent pacemaker. I was working in the homeland of the first 'permanent' pacemaker, manufactured by Joseph Lucas in an engineering company associated with the Queen Elizabeth Hospital in Birmingham. Insertion of the pacemaker was relatively simple. A surgeon made a small incision in the chest wall over the heart, and electrodes, inserted into the muscle of the left ventricle, were attached to a magnetic ring, which was then embedded in the muscle of the chest wall. When the wound was closed, an external magnetic ring, equalling in size the subcutaneous ring, was applied to the skin, and wires from this electrode were connected to a battery-powered box worn on a waist belt. There were simple controls to switch on the device and set the heart rate, and there was an indicator to alert the patient to the need for replacement batteries.[21] The Lucas pacemaker restored many to a life free from recurrent Stokes-Adams attacks, and it also removed the ever-present threat of sudden death.

However, one delightful patient, Bernard, found an alternative use for his pacemaker, which has gone unrecorded in scientific literature. After several episodes of loss of consciousness attributable to Stokes-Adams attacks, Bernard was fitted with a Lucas pacemaker. At his follow-up appointment, he confided to me that his pacemaker did more than prevent loss of consciousness. In his local pub, placing his pacemaker on the bar, he explained the workings of it to a curious ensemble. An inebriated wag suggested that he turn it off to see what would happen. Bernard demurred until a wager of one pint for every minute the device was 'off' was agreed upon. He was now able to drink gratis, thanks to his pacemaker. I advised him to keep the period of switching off the pacemaker as short as possible and to have one trusted (and reasonably sober) accomplice on hand to switch it on should he lose consciousness. This advice might be justly criticized – if Bernard collapsed in the pub with the pacemaker off, a justice presiding over a posthumous action by his family would disapprove of my connivance in his escapade. But the intimacy between a doctor and a patient sometimes reaches far beyond the restrictive dictates of medicine, science and the law.

CCUs allowed patients to survive the complications of a heart attack that would have been fatal. However, they often became laboratories for experimentation in the days before informed consent and ethical approval for studies. Looking back on a publication of which I was a co-author, describing the use of a new drug for patients in shock after a heart attack, I am struck by two features: firstly, there is no mention of consent by the patients; and secondly, even though the drug seems to have had little benefit, the article was accepted for publication.[22] Maurice Pappworth vehemently attacked poorly controlled research in his iconoclastic book, *Human Guinea Pigs*, which led to the principle of consent by patients and the overseeing of research by hospital ethics committees. I admit I was guilty of what Pappworth so ably and rightly denounced.[23]

Mackinnon trained me in the procedure of cardiac catheterisation that allowed visualization of the cardiac chambers to assess the performance of the heart and, more importantly, to assess the damage done to the valves by rheumatic fever. Soon obstructive lesions of the coronary arteries could be visualized, and shortly afterwards, coronary artery bypass surgery (CABS), which enabled a surgeon to take a vein from the leg to bypass the obstructed coronary artery, became commonplace. Unfortunately, CABS was not subjected to the critical assessment that new drugs were given before approval for patient use. The result was that some cardiologists and cardiac surgeons performed CABS without discretion, motivated more by personal gain than by scientific evidence of benefit from the operation. This practice, whereby doctors select patients for procedures from which they will benefit financially, or which will benefit institutions, continues to bedevil medicine and is a contributing factor in the spiralling cost of treatment today.

I enjoyed my training in cardiology at Dudley Road, but soon it was time for a change. Advised by Mackinnon, I moved northwards as Senior Registrar in the Department of Cardiology at the Manchester Royal Infirmary (MRI), where Mackinnon himself had trained. This was a major teaching hospital with a large cardiological department, but I think it is fair to say it did not achieve international scientific credibility. Geoffrey Wade was the head of the department, assisted by two cardiologists, Geoffrey Howarth and Derek Rowlands. The lack of order in the department was disturbing. On one memorable occasion a frustrated cardiac registrar writing a summary letter for a patient muttered his wish that the cardiologist in charge be stricken with a heart attack to which another registrar responded with delightful British wit: 'His system wouldn't have the ability to organize the clot!'

I introduced one innovative procedure during my time in the MRI. There were techniques available to obtain a small piece of tissue – a biopsy – from most organs for microscopic examination to assist diagnosis. However, the heart had been an exception until a Japanese cardiologist, Dr Souji Konno, developed the 'Konno bioptome' in 1962. A catheter could be introduced into the heart from a vein in the arm. When wedged against the heart muscle, a small clip operated from the proximal end of the catheter could pinch a piece of tissue that could then be extracted for microscopic examination. When working in gastroenterology I had been impressed by the orderly classification of liver disease made possible by studying liver biopsies: if the same methodology were applied to a group of heart diseases, known as cardiomyopathies, in which the heart muscle becomes diseased and fails to function properly, it might be possible to classify different patterns of muscle disease based on the histology. I now admit that my initial enthusiasm for the histological classification of the cardiomyopathies added little to our understanding of this group of diseases .[24]

During my time in the MRI, I became conscious of my cultural poverty. I attempted to redress this by enrolling with the Open University for a BA, with an emphasis on logic and philosophy. I began to write about the history of medicine, beginning with the group of Victorian doctors who founded 'The Dublin School'. The leaders of this remarkable movement were Robert Graves, William Stokes, Dominic Corrigan, John Cheyne and Robert Adams. The value of their contributions continues to be acknowledged worldwide two centuries later in the eponyms: Stokes-Adams disease, Cheyne-Stokes respiration, Graves' disease, Corrigan's disease and Corrigan's pulse.

Then I made what was undoubtedly a most irresponsible decision. And in all truth, looking back, even with the wisdom of experience, it isn't possible to attribute any sagacity to what I did, least of all excuse the irresponsibility of throwing years of hard work and sacrifice to the winds of chance. I decided to start a new life away from medicine. This incomprehensible decision may have been a symptom of frustration with specialist medicine. Perhaps I had seen too many disillusioned senior registrars, people of promise who would never fulfil their ambition to reach the consultant grade, or if they did, it would be in some godforsaken part of the country. I resolved never to join that queue of disaffected one-time ambitious and hopeful aspirants. I wanted to write.

As Tona and I were driving from Birmingham to Manchester, I expressed my disillusionment with medicine and my growing desire to write. I hankered to return to Kyrenia in Cyprus where I had been a few years earlier. After a night's discussion we decided we would go. I would take a break from medicine and indulge in literary endeavours.

I gave Geoffrey Wade my notice of resignation. He begged me to reconsider but accepted my decision. In Dublin I rationalized the decision with my father, who had reached a stage of disinterest in life and merely said, 'You're old enough to paddle your own canoe.'

I visited my professor and mentor Alan Thompson in the cottage he was restoring in Inch, County Wicklow. As we sat drinking tea from tin mugs in the quietude of this retreat, Alan advised me that if he were to don the mantle of the wise and conventional mentor, he would caution me against going, but accepted too that life without risk of failure would be a dull affair. We parted with a handshake and the promise that I would keep in contact. I did not know then of Thompson's close association with Samuel Beckett. With hindsight, I see a common thread of philosophical thought between these two students from Portora Royal School in Enniskillen. Thompson saw the likely outcome my erratic path augured for my future, but in keeping with Beckett's evaluation of success, he subscribed to a philosophy that espoused having 'the courage to fail'.

As I worked my notice in the MRI, Tona and I prepared for Cyprus and my departure from medicine. We sold our Manchester house at a small profit that would provide support for a time. Then fate intervened. My father became unwell with an undiagnosed illness. I visited him shortly before his death in Hume Street Nursing Home. The visit does not bring back warm memories and when he 'turned to the wall', I failed to recognize his need for comfort. He died without any family member being with him and I have regretted my insensitivity ever since.

I sometimes wonder if my father's death brought a sense of realism to my life. What in my flimsy literary past suggested I could turn to writing as an occupation? Tona and I abandoned the Cyprus plan. I found myself back in Dublin in 1973 as a jobless cardiologist adrift once more on the ocean of academic medicine. Harry Counihan, one of the physicians in the Richmond, advised my mother, *sotto voce*, that my best hope was to apply for a physician post in rural Ireland – a prospect that didn't appeal to me. In August 1973 Tona found the house that was to be our home and we moved into a place of beauty where we lived for forty-five years, overlooking the ever-changing sea of Seapoint.[25]

Small job opportunities kept the wolf from the door. Stephen Doyle, a physician at the Richmond, relinquished a sessional commitment to Our Lady's Hospital in Navan to me. Harry O'Flanagan, Registrar in the RCSI, appointed me as editor for the College journal. I became Clinical Supervisor of the Membership Examination for the Royal College of Physicians. Then Mervyn (Muff) Abrahamson, who was Professor of Pharmacology and Therapeutics at the

RCSI and Consultant Physician to the Richmond Hospital, resigned his position in deference to his wife's wish to emigrate to Israel. I was appointed in a locum capacity to replace him in both positions. Taking over Abrahamson's duties in the Richmond did not present me with any difficulties, but the professorial obligation to give an hourly lecture each evening of the academic term obliged me to study the pharmacology and therapeutic use of drugs. It was a challenge, but it was also helpful in that it alerted me to the use of new drugs.

I was happy to be back in my alma mater. The Richmond was different to other hospitals in that it had a fascinating cultural personality.[26] Lunch was always interesting. Here under the kind and watchful eye of Mary Byrnes, who oversaw our epicurean requirements with motherly affection, eclectic conversations erupted with dramatic spontaneity. The rhythm and cadence of the ribald and irreverent ballad 'Bunga Bing'[27] written by an Irish doctor might vie for critical attention with Wagner's *Valkyrie* in Bayreuth, as recounted by the music-loving anaesthetist, Johnny Conroy. While Hugh Staunton expounded on fly-fishing in the west of Ireland, Paddy Bofin might be heard marvelling at the semantic ingeniousness of a senior garda's pronouncement that the city was being overrun, not so much by prostitutes, but by 'little whoreens'. David Bouchier-Hayes, with whom I rekindled our schoolboy friendship, and who was now establishing himself as an innovative surgeon with a flair for research, was a delightful raconteur; his mischievous humour bode poorly for those who became the butt of his wit. Harold Browne, a surgeon with a gentle outlook on life, might muse on the oddity of a patient studying, with the assistance of a torch and mirror, the healing of his rectum without its haemorrhoids. Alan Thompson could provide any reference to classical literature that might be wanting, and as if these literary nuances were not enough, there was Jack Widdess, physician, historian, man of letters, bibliophile and mentor to aspiring historians, who was the director of the hospital's biochemistry lab. Jack's laconic humour often astounded his listeners. He never regarded himself as 'a proper doctor', but this did not deter him from undertaking an occasional locum for his neighbouring GP. When on a beauteous spring day he was informed that a titled notable had collapsed while tending to his beloved roses and that his presence was urgently sought, Jack took the long coast road to admire the sun upon the billow, the coots and the swans, thereby acknowledging that the Creator would not be gainsaid.

As hospitals in Dublin (or anywhere for that matter) go, few can match the Richmond's contribution to literature. Oliver St John Gogarty – an ear, nose and throat surgeon – had the audacity (or contempt) to confront the mores of a censorious public with ribald prose, wit and poetry. His poem 'Ringsend' opens with the strident declaration:

> I will live in Ringsend
> With a red-headed whore,
> And the fanlight gone in
> Where it lights the hall-door[28]

Daragh Smith, who graced the Richmond in the 1930s, left a bawdy glimpse of an irreverent age in his *Dissecting Room Ballads*. And then there was John Pollock, a pathologist who, along with poetry and criticism, wrote commendable and gently humorous novels. I never came to befriend Pollock, much to my regret – the age difference was too great, but I was one of a small group of students gathered in his museum of pathological specimens in the Whitworth Hospital where he demonstrated the cruel assault of illness on various organs with a placid timbre of tone interspersed with references to poetry and literature.

It wasn't long before decision time came again. I was presented with a dilemma. In 1976 two consultant positions became vacant. The locum post I was occupying in the Richmond was advertised for a 'cardiologist trained in performing catheter studies', and the nearby sister teaching hospital, the Charitable Infirmary, advertised for a physician with a special interest in cardiology. I had been trained in coronary angiography in the UK and could have refreshed this skill, but when I considered the prospect of performing angiographic studies in a catheter laboratory for the rest of my career, I decided I would prefer the challenge of treating cardiovascular disease in its totality. I submitted my application to the Charitable Infirmary.

Except for John Fielding, the staff in the Charitable Infirmary were unknown to me, although the Professor of Medicine, Billy O'Dwyer, professed a close friendship with my mother. On the day of the interview, I waited in the hall with apprehension. I worried that my appearance might count against me, having been advised by Fielding to shave off my beard, which I refused to do. I was an experienced contender for hospital appointments, but nothing prepared me for what lay ahead.

The interview had such an air of unreality that the cinematic powers of Ealing Studios would have been at a loss to capture the atmosphere. I was ushered into a large room and directed to a chair that stood in isolation on one side of a wide boardroom table opposite a dozen seated men comprising the medical and surgical staff of the hospital. Their place at the table was decreed by seniority so that the most senior physician and surgeon were seated at the centre with diminishing rank dictating order towards the periphery on either side – da Vinci might have thought the scene familiar but for the absence of bread and wine. Beyond this table more men leaned against ionic pillars that gave the Victorian room an indeterminate dimension. These men, I would later learn, were the governors of the hospital. They comprised local traders and publicans and they chatted among themselves, smoking and drinking from china cups. Two nuns scurried to and fro with coffee, which (as I would also later learn) was laced liberally from a bottle of Green Spot whiskey closeted discreetly in their vestments. Since there were only six appointments (three surgeons and three physicians) and given a working lifespan of say twenty years, appointments to the staff under the Charter granted by George III in 1792 were rare. The selection of a senior physician in accordance with the revered charter was a circumstance of importance that merited a large turnout.

The interview was led by the senior physician and professor of medicine, W.F. O'Dwyer, who favoured another candidate. He questioned me on the practice of clinical medicine, and having demonstrated my training in cardiology, he went on to demean the facilities that would be at my disposal for cardiological practice should I be successful; he stressed that this deficiency would leave me with no alternative but to make exorbitant demands on the already depleted hospital exchequer. Fielding had tipped me off to this ploy, so I stayed with the theme of cardiovascular medicine being a growing discipline that needed imaginative management by a well-trained general physician. I would secure whatever financial support I required from the pharmaceutical industry and grant-awarding bodies to develop research without having to seek hospital support. A governor stepped forward from the background cabal, cigarette in hand, to ask me if I was aware of the hospital's august history. I cited the names of the founding surgeons and summarized their laudable mission. I outlined the remarkable contributions to medicine by two former members of the staff, Robert Adams and Dominic Corrigan, who were remembered today by the eponyms Stokes-Adams attack and Corrigan's Disease, adding that should I be appointed to the position Corrigan had once occupied with such distinction, I would do all I could to emulate his outstanding contributions to clinical medicine.

I was offered the appointment of Senior Consultant Physician in Cardiology to the Charitable Infirmary, better known as Jervis Street Hospital – or simply

'The Jerv' by Dubliners. The appointment also carried the position of Visiting Consultant Cardiologist to the James Connolly Memorial Hospital in Blanchardstown. Harold Browne, in the Richmond, well-known for his caustic turn of phrase, expressed sadness at my departure while also giving vent to his jaundiced view of The Jerv: 'Well, Eoin, you are now off to join The Lavender Hill Mob.' I was soon to learn he had a point. If example was needed to give substance to this allegation, it was to be found in the persona of Peter Flood, a much-disliked surgeon, who deserted surgery for the priesthood but only after acquiring so many postgraduate university qualifications that he earned the accolade of possessing 'more degrees than a thermometer without the same capacity for registering warmth'. In attempting to acquaint myself with the history of my new hospital, I visited Dom Peter Flood in Ealing Abbey to determine if the myth was a reality.[29]

The Jerv was a run-down hospital with little going for it except its illustrious history. The Charitable Infirmary was the first voluntary hospital in Ireland and Great Britain. It was opened in 1718 by six Dublin surgeons appalled by the conditions afflicting the sick poor of the city. Diminutive and humble as the institute was, it had a profound influence on the social history of Dublin, which had been without a hospital since Henry VIII applied his act for the suppression of monasteries to Ireland. The altruism of the founding doctors of the Charitable Infirmary ignited the voluntary hospital movement.[30]

If the facilities in the Richmond were below standard, there were no provisions whatsoever for cardiology in The Jerv. A small room already occupied by the ECG technician now served as her office and mine. My future as a cardiologist was dependent on acquiring financial support outside the hospital. History once again taught me there is nothing new under the sun. If Handel, who had performed *Messiah* in Dublin's Fishamble Street in 1742, was persuaded to allocate the proceeds to the Charitable Infirmary, then I too could appeal to benefactors.[31] I turned first to the College of Surgeons, which funded the purchase of a Portakabin that we placed on the last piece of garden in the hospital.

Next, I approached the pharmaceutical industry, which provided sponsorship for nursing and research staff. John Fielding, who would later become professor of medicine, supported me in every way possible, and Des O'Riordan, an anaesthetist, agreed to divide the Intensive Care Unit (ICU) to provide me with beds for a CCU. The sister in charge of the ICU, Noreen Rafferty, gave me the necessary nursing backing and proved to be a loyal colleague. Paddy Collins, the ebullient professor of surgery, supported me in my struggles with the hospital board. O'Dwyer, the professor of medicine, did all he could to make life difficult for me, but, importantly, I persuaded the board to fund a cardiac registrar. In response to the ad for this position, a doctor named Leslie Lam presented himself to persuade me to give him the job because he believed I could tutor him to pass the membership exam, without which he would be unable to return to his native Singapore. Thus began a relationship that has lasted to the present day. Leslie was one of the best registrars I ever had. Between us we developed a rudimentary cardiac department. Leslie's willingness to share clinical responsibilities allowed me to develop the department's research activities. He passed his membership exam and returned to Singapore where he developed his own cardiac department and went on to be physician to the Sultan of Brunei.[32]

I was also fortunate in enlisting the nursing assistance of Fiansia Mee and the statistical and computer expertise of Neil Atkins, each of whom would play an important role in research into hypertension. I continued working in the Charitable Infirmary until it was amalgamated with the Richmond as Beaumont Hospital.

When Beaumont Hospital opened on 29 November 1987, I began a seventeen-year association that ranks as the unhappiest of all my hospital appointments. Things went badly from the outset. I visited the administrative officers a year before the opening to discuss the historical background to the naming of the wards. My views on the appropriate nomenclature for wards in a non-sectarian hospital were at variance with the popular religion of the land, which was upheld with conviction by the *in loco* administration. But this was not to be my only disagreement on matters of nomenclature. The Department of Health sought my advice on the naming of the hospital and the design of the crest. I suggested 'The Corrigan Hospital at Beaumont'.[33] Interestingly, two reasons were put forward by the Department of Health for declining this proposal. The first was that Corrigan, although Catholic, declined the Chair of Medicine in 1855 at the newly founded Catholic University in Cecilia Street because, as a Liberal MP in Gladstone's government, he opposed sectarian education at university level. More than a century later, the elephantine memory of the ardently religious civil service saw it as preferable to name the new hospital after the first Viscount of Beaumont, whose only claim to fame was that his son had been cashiered out of the British army for refusing to allow Catholics into it.

The second objection to the Corrigan name was mooted only in hushed conversation by those in the know that a more worthy recipient – Charles

Haughey – might need commemoration at some not-too-distant date. Beside this perverse logic, it had also escaped the notice of the governmental savants that a hospital in Michigan boasted the same name, but in this instance to honour the memory of a famous American physician, William Beaumont. These nomenclative mishaps could be reversed, of course; the hospital could be renamed The Corrigan University Hospital at Beaumont. To do so would not only honour a Dubliner who had contributed immensely to science and humanitarianism but would also convey to international medicine a justifiable claim on excellence in both the practice and science of medicine.

Should Beaumont Hospital ever excite future historical assessment, it is likely that the incompetent preparation preceding the amalgamation of the two hospitals might be overlooked. A substantial team of administrators, which included a CEO and a director of nursing, had been seconded to the hospital years in advance of its opening with the objective of anticipating the logistical difficulties of merging the two hospitals. Their failure to do so resulted in chaos. On the opening day, ambulances bearing hundreds of patients and two-thousand staff arrived at the hospital. The primary concern of the medical staff was to ensure the safety of the patients in the face of a non-existent infrastructure, whereas the primary concern of the administrative staff was to label the doctors and nurses immediately on arrival, rather than have them attend patients who, in the absence of charts, a dysfunctional telephonic and bleep system, were deprived of the basic support mechanisms for safe hospital care. I remember being particularly concerned about patients on warfarin, who were dependent on laboratory verification and efficient communication to determine the optimal dosage of the drug.

The chaos of patient management was only one aspect of this dysfunctional hospital. There was the added mayhem created by the dismantling of the internal governance structures, such as a medical board and an ethics committee. In effect, a system that had been tried and modified over the 250 years of the voluntary hospital movement in Ireland was rendered defunct. As a result, the Department of Health, which had never run a hospital without the support of the voluntary hospital infrastructure, was adrift without the procedures needed to ensure patient safety and staff morale. Eventually, a delegation of consultants (of which I was a member) visited the Department of Health and left the minister in no doubt that if urgent measures were not taken, Beaumont Hospital, touted as the pride of Ireland's hospital service, would sink as surely as the *Titanic*. The outcome was that Seamus Dawson was replaced by Michael McLoone in February 1988 to take over management of the hospital.

McLoone's priority was to restore staff morale. He replaced the defunct committees and gave staff the ability to express grievances. Furthermore, he was receptive to ideas for innovation and improvement. He steadied the sinking ship and was making good progress when he discovered that if his remit to establish a centre of excellence was to be realized, a rolling budget over a five-year period was required rather than the customary annual allocation of funds. The Department of Health ignored McLoone's threatened resignation, with the result that he departed Beaumont and whatever hope the hospital had of achieving excellence departed with him. The failure of Beaumont to achieve the stated ambition of becoming a 'centre of excellence' cannot be blamed entirely on poor management. Unfortunately, the institute was also haunted by 'consultant hubris'. This phenomenon is common in the Irish healthcare system, but it was given undue presence in Beaumont because some remarkably egotistical personalities were faced with the diminution of their hitherto unbridled power.

I was glad to depart Beaumont Hospital in 2004. It was an unhappy hospital, and whatever misgivings I had about the many hospitals I had served – the Richmond, the Charitable Infirmary, the Rotunda, Monkstown Hospital, Our Lady's Hospital in Navan, the James Connolly Memorial Hospital and the City of Dublin Skin and Cancer Hospital, their dominant ethos was to make sick people well again. Beaumont, by contrast, was continuously involved in controversy and selfishly motivated bickering, partly because it was managed by inexperienced people who did not know the meaning of the word 'excellence'.

However, there were positive aspects: wonderful nursing staff, among whom Dolly Coyne stands supreme; with my cardiological colleagues, John Horgan and Tom Gumbrielle, we provided a good service to patients with cardiac disease and my childhood friend David Bouchier-Hayes provided exemplary support for patients with vascular disease; the loyal staff in the Blood Pressure Unit provided a service based on well-founded research; and then there was the privilege of caring for many thousands of patients with cardiovascular disease, each of whom in their own ways taught me something about life and, unfortunately betimes, death, and who helped to make me a better doctor. Many students also taught me more than I ever taught them. And lest they be forgotten, there were the chaplains, nuns, porters, telephonists and other ancillary staff members who put frightened patients and relatives at ease with their welcoming warmth.

5. The Wider World of Medicine

The man of science is too often a person who has exchanged his soul for a formula.
W.B. Yeats, 'Poetry and Science in Folklore', *Uncollected Prose* (1890)

As a cardiologist in the Charitable Infirmary, and with paltry facilities, I had to decide on a research topic that would benefit patients and attract funding. Having considered the many facets of cardiovascular medicine for research opportunities, I decided on hypertension, which I saw as the major underlying cause of heart disease and stroke sweeping across the world.

My interest in hypertension began in Dudley Road Hospital with the publication of two papers on treating hypertension with a new class of drugs known as beta-blockers.[1] These papers led to an invitation in 1975 to a conference in Malta entitled 'Hypertension – Its Nature and Treatment.'[2] I was alone on the bus from Valletta airport to the hotel when a man in a grubby raincoat asked if he could sit beside me. He was Sir George Pickering, then the most influential scientist in the world on this illness.[3] He enquired with interest about my research ambitions. We were destined to meet the following morning when he would chair a session at which I was to present a talk on the benefit of beta-blocking drugs.

The meeting didn't start well. Sir George arrived late, shaking his watch, conveying that his belatedness could be blamed on an unreliable chronometer. He invited me to the podium. As I signalled to the projectionist at the back of the small room, I heard the ominous but unmistakable sound of slides cascading from a carousel to the floor. Sir George, anxious not to delay matters, addressed the audience with the words I have never forgotten: 'Well now, O'Brien faces the horror we all dread – he is on his own, slide-less. Proceed, O'Brien.' Thanks to the sleepless night that usually precedes such occasions, I had not only learnt each slide but had copied them onto prompt cards. This saved me, and I successfully delivered my paper. Later, in commending my presentation, Pickering warned against relying on technology. I did not fulfil my ambition to work in Pickering's Oxford unit, but he would later advise me on the course of my research.

In Malta I was also fortunate to meet William Kannel, director of the Framingham Study in Massachusetts, which had commenced in 1948 when the citizens of Framingham agreed to participate in a study that has influenced the management of cardiovascular disease for four generations.[4] Kannel warned at the conference that the mistreatment of hypertension was causing preventable strokes and heart attacks. Returning from Malta, I decided to focus my research on hypertension.

When Kevin O'Malley was appointed Professor of Pharmacology and Therapeutics at the RCSI in 1978, we joined forces to establish the Blood Pressure Unit (BPU) – one of the first centres in Europe dedicated to researching the causes of high blood pressure.[5] The BPU studied methods of diagnosis, measurement techniques, assessment of management strategies and drug treatment (particularly in the elderly) and created public awareness of hypertension. Convinced that the study of hypertension was dependent on analysing patient data, I purchased the first personal computer, the BBC Microcomputer (known affectionately as the Beeb) in 1978. We designed software to manage blood-pressure measurements and data from over 50,000 hypertensive patients has since been entered into this database, now one of the largest in the world.

O'Malley concentrated on the treatment of high blood pressure in the elderly, and I explored new methods for measuring blood pressure, particularly the measurement of blood pressure over twenty-four hours. In the 1980s high blood pressure was considered an inevitable consequence of ageing. In a review co-authored by O'Malley and me in the *New England Journal of Medicine*, we highlighted the need for research to determine if elderly patients with hypertension should be treated.[6] Such questions can be answered only by studying large numbers of patients – we recognized that future research depended on sharing our skills and resources with other units. This approach led to the BPU participating in collaborative trials with other hypertension centres worldwide.

In 1978 the BPU drew attention to the importance of accurate measurement of blood pressure in a series of papers in the *British Medical Journal* entitled 'The ABC of Blood Pressure Measurement'.[7] Until then, the method of measuring a variable phenomenon on which the diagnosis, treatment and prognosis of hypertension is dependent was taken for granted. Jan Staessen, a young scientist in Louvain, involved in organizing a major European study of hypertension in the elderly, shared an empirical scepticism about scientific claims based on traditional methods of blood-pressure measurement; we continue to question to this day the foundation on which the science of hypertension is dependent.

The technique of blood-pressure measurement has evolved over three centuries since the Reverend Stephen Hales demonstrated, in 1733, that blood rose to a height of 8ft 3in in a glass tube placed in the artery of a horse.[8] The history of blood-pressure measurement is intriguing, but the doctor who introduced the clinical method of measuring it, Nikolai Korotkoff, is the most fascinating part of the story in that we know so little about him and his humanitarian idealism.

My quest for information on Korotkoff brought me into correspondence with the Canadian cardiologist Harold Segall, who had written biographical essays on him. I met Segall in Ghent in 1981, where we were presenting papers to a meeting on ambulatory blood pressure monitoring. I was impressed by his gentle, persuasive personality, and we formed a friendship that lasted until his death in 1990 at the age of ninety-two.[9] After this encounter in Ghent, I became even more fascinated by Korotkoff, and Segall had managed to trace his son, Dr Serge Korotkoff, who had written a biography of his father. When I attended the World Congress of Cardiology in Moscow in 1982, Segall arranged for me to meet Korotkoff in St Petersburg. However, just as I was about to leave for St Petersburg, I received a telegram informing me of his death and I have since failed to obtain the biography of his father which, to the best of my knowledge, remains unpublished and we still have only brief details on the life of this remarkable man.[10]

As I continued examining methods of blood-pressure measurement, Sir George Pickering once again influenced my research. I was intrigued by his method of measuring blood pressure over twenty-four hours, but its use was limited because a small catheter had to be inserted into the brachial artery and left throughout the day and night. Pickering advised me to contact NASA, where a device for measuring blood pressure in astronauts was in development. I travelled to San Francisco where the company manufacturing the device was located and returned with two Remler devices that could measure blood pressure every half-hour away from the disturbing hospital environment.

The BPU performed the first non-invasive ambulatory blood-pressure measurement in 1980. A paper published in 1985 made a prescient observation that in many patients with high blood pressure measured using the conventional hospital technique, the daytime ambulatory blood pressure was significantly lower.[11] Had I been in a serendipitous mood, I would have attributed the phenomenon to 'white-coat hypertension', in which an elevated blood pressure falls to normal levels once the patient is away from the medical environment. However, the discovery of this condition would await the succinct description by Thomas Pickering, Sir George's son, in 1988.[12]

It was not long before devices capable of measuring blood pressure over 24 hours were developed. In a letter to *The Lancet* in 1988, data from the BPU showed that patients with a reduction in night-time blood pressure had a significantly better prognosis than those without. As a result, the terms 'dippers' and 'non-dippers' entered the medical nomenclature.[13]

The BPU next began to examine the accuracy of the devices used to measure blood pressure. We showed that many devices were inaccurate and, surprisingly, that the two 'gold standard' devices in clinical research were also inaccurate – a damning indictment of science. Aware of the reaction that would ensue, I asked Ronán Conroy, a statistician and epidemiologist of international stature, to examine the data.[14] I also invited Tony Lever, head of the Department of Medicine and Therapeutics at the University of Glasgow, an acknowledged leader of hypertension research, to visit the BPU to examine our experimental methodology.[15] Lever's visit was a highlight in the history of the BPU. His intellectual versatility could turn from a discourse on the obliquity of colour in a Bonnard painting to solving a statistical conundrum in a scientific table. Our deliberations raised doubts about the fallibility of some international research by distinguished scientists. If the devices used in many research studies were inaccurate, the conclusions of numerous papers published in medical journals must be at best questionable and at worst flawed. What impact would a reassessment of this have on scientific issues, such as the effectiveness of drugs to lower blood pressure? Unfortunately, we'll never know since the analysis hasn't been done!

As the BPU continued to advocate for accurate measurement of blood pressure through publication of research, I knew it was necessary also to influence international regulatory and consumer bodies such as the British Standards Institution (BSI), the Food and Drug Administration (FDA), the International Organization for Standardization (ISO) and the World Health Organisation (WHO). I joined the committees of these bodies and made friends in unrelated disciplines.[16] However, most of the personnel were focused on selling as many devices as possible, regardless of their accuracy. I explored ways of making information on device accuracy available to the consumer market, as well as the medical profession, using website technology. This was difficult because the principles governing commercial behaviour were often incompatible with scientific principles. However, with my colleague and friend George Stergiou, we established the STRIDE BP initiative in 2018 as a not-for-profit endeavour and this website is now providing information on accuracy to consumers worldwide.[17]

In 1968 I voiced my misgivings about the fragmentation of the practice of cardiovascular medicine to Richard Horton, the editor of *The Lancet*. This led me to change the remit of the original BPU, which I renamed the Arterial Disease Assessment Prevention and Treatment (ADAPT) Centre. The rationale for this broader remit was the realization that patients suffering from cardiovascular disease should be managed according to a common strategy directed at the arterial organ, regardless of the specialist to whom they presented.[18]

On the day of my compulsory retirement from Beaumont in December 2004, aged sixty-five, I had an ignominious meeting with the administration headed by the CEO, Liam Duffy, and the cardiologists. My offer to continue overseeing my research projects was rejected. Instead, they proposed that my hypertension research should be managed by the cardiologists. This meant that my twenty-five years of research was in turmoil. Fortunately, Patricia McCormack, a loyal colleague whose name appears on many BPU publications, agreed to take charge in an interim period. Then Desmond Fitzgerald, who was Vice-President for Research at UCD, and who had worked in the BPU for many years, arranged for my appointment to the Chair of Molecular Pharmacology at the Conway Institute for Biomolecular and Biomedical Research in UCD. Laurent Perret (President of the Scientific Committee of the Servier Research Group in Paris, a company with which the BPU had performed collaborative research since 1979), endowed a chair for me at UCD. One of my protégés, Eamon Dolan, who had applied his expertise successfully to study the role of hypertension in causing stroke in Addenbrooke's Hospital in Cambridge and later in the James Connolly

Hospital in Dublin, assisted me in producing collaborative studies based on the Dublin database on hypertension. In Beaumont Hospital, which I had left, Alice Stanton, supported by a band of loyal nurses and secretaries, ensured that the BPU continued to provide care to patients with high blood pressure. Aware that there was turmoil in my research, my international friends in science provided much-needed support so that I could contribute my expertise to collaborative scientific projects across the world.

The research undertaken in the BPU and ADAPT Centre may be assessed from the hundreds of papers published in peer-reviewed journals and by international presentations. It is apparent from the diversity of co-authors how dependent the unit was on collaborative research and on many sources of financial support.[19] But successes were overshadowed by our inability to implement procedures and policies based on scientific logic. A major failing was being unable to persuade doctors to recognize the fallibility of blood-pressure measurement, or, put another way, my inability to convince them.

Why, after writing hundreds of papers, was I unable to alert the world to this empirical reality? How do international bodies (such as the WHO) base their recommendations on inaccurate data? How can regulatory bodies (such as the FDA) recommend devices that have not been subjected to validation studies? How can scientific journals publish research ignoring measurement methodology? How can we counter the manufacturing and pharmaceutical industries who indirectly (and directly) fatten the purses of their shareholders based on two numbers: the systolic and diastolic blood pressures generated by inaccurate measurement methodologies? How can clinical researchers trained in scientific methods continue to uphold inaccurate measurement techniques? How would a gullible public who regard scientists as omnipotent and trustworthy react to such shortcomings?

It could be argued that my time as a cardiologist should have been devoted to caring for patients with heart disease. But research informs the clinician's mind and allows critical awareness of the procedures developed to overcome illness. This said, research at consultant level calls for personal sacrifice: the fiscal attraction of private practice must be sublimated in favour of research to learn more about illness and, by doing so, attempt to improve its management. The bureaucracy of research, which has become onerous, should not be allowed to overwhelm the spirit of enquiry. Teaching hospitals should provide a research secretariat to lessen this necessary burden of clinical research. Research should become the rule rather than the exception. Patients are aware that they benefit by being enrolled in clinical trials. If government agencies such as Enterprise Ireland, the Industrial Development Authority and the Department of Health provided financial assistance to establish and harness data from registries and then used their marketing expertise, Ireland could become an international mecca for research. The creation of an 'island of research', with all patients enrolled in clinical studies, would bring structured care to patients, and Ireland could become a leader in the acquisition of collaborative research funding, as well as attracting funding from the pharmacological and technological industries for scientific studies.

Doctors have always had a unique opportunity to appreciate how illness affects populations in poverty-stricken countries, but until recently humanitarian issues have not been on medical schools' curricula. In 1992 I was introduced to Kevin Cahill, professor of tropical medicine in the RCSI. He founded the Center for International Humanitarian Co-operation (CIHC) in New York to promote healing and peace in countries shattered by natural disasters, armed conflicts and ethnic violence. I joined the board of CIHC and met people willing to give their time to encourage humanitarian assistance in such countries.[20] Among these were Paul Hamlyn and his wife, Helen, a woman of remarkable enterprise and energy, both of whom became close friends. Paul was a publisher and benefactor who established the Paul Hamlyn Foundation, one of the UK's largest independent grant-giving organizations, as a focus for his charitable interests. When I joined the CIHC, I wanted to add momentum to the demand for an international land-mine ban. I wrote essays on the horror of these wretched weapons.[21] I visited the Sawai Man Singh Hospital in Jaipur at Paul Hamlyn's request to look at ways of increasing the use of the 'Jaipur limb' among amputees in mine-stricken countries: this ingenious prosthesis was simple and inexpensive and could withstand the rugged conditions in countries devastated by land mines. In 1996 I made a presentation on 'The Diplomatic Implications of Emerging Diseases' in the UN with the Secretary General, Kofi Annan, chairing a symposium on preventive diplomacy – it is worth mentioning that had the recommendations of that symposium been enacted, global healthcare services would have been better prepared for COVID-19.[22]

From studying the history of medicine, I understood there were times when the establishment should be scrutinized, and that critical appraisal was most effective when instigated from within. It was fortunate, therefore, that Michael

O'Donnell, the flamboyant editor of *World Medicine*, asked me to contribute to his magazine. O'Donnell challenged orthodox medicine, especially the General Medical Council (GMC), the body that governs the profession.[23] *World Medicine* probably did more for medicine in the period when it flourished (1965–82) than the long-established *British Medical Journal* and *The Lancet* which were, by comparison, conservative and dull. Even the editor of the *British Medical Journal*, Stephen Lock, wrote: 'Not to have read Michael O'Donnell's *World Medicine* was to have been incomplete as a doctor.'[24] O'Donnell introduced me to Richard Leech, another polemical writer, who wrote a regular feature, 'Doctor in the Wings'.[25] And so I began life as a medical journalist writing, mostly anonymously, for *World Medicine*.[26]

In 1970, Lock, then a staff editor of the *British Medical Journal*, recruited me to join a group of staff reporters including Bill Whimster, Bertie Wood (who could provide the social and family background of any notable in Scottish medicine) and Jim Petrie (destined to become a major influence in academic medicine in Scotland).[27] We travelled to many BMA meetings in close friendship over a five-year period under the watchful eye of either Stephen Lock, or Richard Smith, then assistant editors of the *British Medical Journal*. The format of reportage on the meetings we attended was rigid, with a pedantic obsession to ensure that the prose was emotively sterile and devoid of any utterance that might betray the writer's personality. If we tried to sneak in a mischievous sentence, it was edited out before the handwritten copy was sent to London for typesetting. A notable example of the rigid style of reportage was the BMA Clinical Meeting in Kingston, Jamaica, in April 1974; despite this, my report to the *British Medical Journal* has a curious historic resonance in reporting the contribution of Michael DeBakey, a renowned cardiac surgeon:

> After studying 10,000 coronary arteriograms over 15 years, he considered that the patterns of the disease could now be seen in two ways. Firstly, occlusive disease could affect the larger arteries leaving the distal ones unimpaired; this could be relieved by operation, such as venous bypass graft or by endarterectomy … Secondly, patients differed in the rate at which occlusive lesions progressed – though in only 25% of patients was the progression rapid. Turning to risk factors, in his series about 80% of the patients had smoked, 40% were hypertensive, 40% had abnormalities of lipoprotein metabolism, and 15% had diabetes.

Given this was in 1974, cardiologists today would agree that this was a prescient summary of cardiovascular disease.

The Jamaica meeting puts me in mind of an amusing incident. The editor of the *British Medical Journal* at the time was Martin Ware, who gave me the impression that neither dark-skinned men nor the Irish occupied positions of esteem in his scheme of international order. To fulfil his obligation of gratitude to his coterie of journalists, he led us to the Blue Mountain Inn, a renowned establishment near Kingston, where a black uniformed doorman refused Ware admission because, since he had no jacket, his attire was deemed inappropriate. An insult to imperial propriety was avoided when the beaming janitor graciously provided a blazer for the abashed editor, and I, the Irishman, was able to make good his necktie deficiency by proffering the one serving to keep my trousers at waist level. All in all, these little travesties aside, the evening progressed splendidly, albeit with the ever-present risk of an unseemly exposé by the Irish reporter as the wine flowed beneath a tropical sky.

These overseas meetings allowed me to explore the cultural and medical aspects of other countries. At the East Mediterranean Medical Congress in Cyprus in 1972, I visited the seaside town of Kyrenia. The medical highlight of the congress was the clinical presentation of six patients with leprosy who could have been cured with dapsone at a minute cost.[28] But the cultural highlight was the beauty of Bellapais Abbey, where Lawrence Durrell had written *Bitter Lemons*. Despite abandoning my decision to live in Kyrenia as writer, I still think frequently about this place of serenity and beauty today.

I contributed many editorials to the *British Medical Journal*, written anonymously, as was then customary. Stephen Lock relished pithy titles and if they drew on literature – as did two of my contributions, 'Or in the heart or in the head' and 'Will no one tell me what she sings?' – so much the better. However, when I submitted an editorial inspired by the death of a French bishop in a brothel with the title 'The bishop in the bordello', prurient editorship modified it to 'Coitus and coronaries' with all reference to the libidinous prelate removed. In 1975 Lock commissioned a series of articles to run as a *Letter from Dublin* to give readers in Britain a flavour of medical and related happenings in Ireland.

Shortly after I returned to Dublin, Harry Counihan, the editor of the *Irish Medical Journal*, invited me to write editorials and later commissioned a series of articles under the designation 'Kincoran Opinion'. I was appointed editor of the *Journal of the Irish Colleges of Physicians and Surgeons* in 1973 and of the *Irish Medical Journal* in 1986. In both journals I sought to display art related to medicine by using a painting or photograph on the cover linked to an article in the issue. As well as the scientific articles, which are the raison d'être of clinical journals, I encouraged articles on the history of medicine and the role of the humanities and humanitarian considerations in the medical curriculum.

I soon learned that my editorial comments could evoke vehement reaction from the profession. An editorial entitled 'What Is a Professor?' owed its existence to an unusual event that took place in Dublin in 1979.[29] The pharmaceutical company Astra endowed two chairs in cardiology in UCD. To mark the occasion, a lavish jamboree was arranged in the Berkeley Court Hotel. Unfortunately, a contingent of dignitaries from the cardiological establishment in Britain was delayed and the welcoming gathering, drawn from the highest reaches of the profession in Ireland, imbibed more than was judicious for the occasion. When we were seated for dinner, Walter Somerville,[30] the then editor of the *British Heart Journal*, noted that the inebriation greeting the sober contingent from Britain wasn't confined to the guests; a waiter was dispensing soup liberally on the carpet as he pirouetted from table to table. Hastily, Somerville wrote on his place card: 'My dear fellow, you have had a little too much to drink and would be well advised to go home.' Picking it up without reading it, the waiter waddled off and mistakenly dropped the message on Professor (later Sir) Colin Dollery's plate who, the story goes, was not amused.

During the evening, I expressed the view that the endowment of two chairs in the small discipline of cardiology in one university demeaned the stature of academic professorships. I was phoned the following morning by one of the endowed professors, Risteárd Mulcahy, telling me I'd be well advised not to air that view in print. Which, of course, I did. Reading this essay now, I could hardly have anticipated that I would add substance to my concluding prediction that 'Dublin would soon earn a reputation similar to that which it once had as a city of "dreadful knights" of now being one of "dismal professors".' I have held no fewer than three chairs and declined a fourth!

Most of my journalistic forays are forgotten but one, surprisingly, has lived on and is still quoted. The enduring popularity of 'Towards Being a Scientific Doctor and the Dangers of the Dublin Disease' is attributable to my description of an affliction that permits the fiscal attraction of private practice to overcome the idealism of scientific research.[31]

In another editorial for the *Journal of the Irish Colleges of Physicians and Surgeons*, I proposed that rather than having two colleges, the RCPI and the RCSI, it made sense to sell the RCPI to the adjoining National Library of Ireland, which needed space. While the article was in press, I was at a dinner in the RCSI and was accosted in the gents by the president (Alan Grant), the treasurer (Bryan Alton) and the registrar (Ciaran Barry), who manned the door to prevent entry by other guests. They told me they found my view was offensive to the RCPI and asked me to withdraw the article, which I refused to do. They declined my invitation to write a response putting forward the College's rebuttal of my proposal.[32]

Worse was to follow. In 1987, as editor of the *Irish Medical Journal*, I wrote an editorial criticizing doctors for withdrawing their services to resolve grievances between the government and the profession, and argued for alternative methods of protest.[33] This opinion offended the Irish Medical Organisation (IMO), which was a trade union and the proprietor of the journal. But rather than dismiss me as editor, they closed the journal on the grounds that it was losing money and reopened it under a new editor months later. The event attracted attention from the *British Medical Journal*, *The Lancet* and the *Journal of the American Association of Medicine*.[34]

Medical journalism took me to Bahrain twice. As editor of the college journal, I attended the first overseas meeting held by the RCSI in 1989 to report the proceedings. One morning, as I sat in the Souk sipping coffee and watching the colourful life around me, an Arab dressed in white, having seen that I was reading *Looking for Dilmun* by Geoffrey Bibby, asked if he could join me. He was Abdulaziz Ali Sowaileh, Superintendent of Archaeology for Bahrain. He invited me to an excavation the next day where I dusted away sand to reveal an exquisite ring, with an agate set in silver, dating back 3000 years.[35]

My interest in Bahrain was rekindled twenty years later when I read a letter from Professor Damian McCormack in *The Irish Times*, deploring the fate of doctors imprisoned in Bahrain when the Arab Spring engulfed the island in February 2011. At the awarding of degrees in Bahrain that year, I was astounded by the failure of the presidents of the RCSI and the RCPI to enquire about forty-seven doctors imprisoned without trial and subjected to torture, some of whom had trained in Dublin and were fellows of the RCSI. I resigned my fellowship of the RCPI in protest. Shortly afterwards, the international human rights organization Front Line Defenders invited me to join a delegation to Bahrain.[36] At the end of our visit we were in no doubt that doctors and medical personnel had been subjected to human-rights abuses. We left Bahrain moved by the gratitude of the medical personnel for our support but embarrassed that we offered so little in the face of their suffering and courage.[37]

I saw medical journalism as a *modus operandi* to challenge establishment doctrine, but the assumption that I would receive reasoned debate from a liberal and educated profession was wrong. Deliberating on these concerns with my friend the barrister Paddy McEntee, I asked how it came to this. Why was I in conflict with the ruling bodies of my profession at a time in my career when such relationships should be tranquil? How did I find myself engaged in controversy with the RCSI of all places – an institution I had respected and eulogized in publications over the years? Why did I find it necessary to resign my fellowship of the RCPI – an honour I worked hard to attain and valued highly? McEntee, with characteristic caution, put my predicament into context in his inimitable way: 'Eoin, you are merely sensing what perhaps you did not have the time or the wisdom to heed hitherto – the corruption of privilege.'[38] How right he was. Institutions are privileged by their influence in society and are further favoured in that they control the fate of their practitioners, who must adhere to establishment conventions. McEntee was also correct in sensing that previously I had not had the wisdom (and courage) to confront the corruption of privilege.

The past is always begging for attention. I had difficulty throwing out a letter or a photograph but, as material accumulated, it was clear I couldn't keep everything. I alleviated the pain of discarding ephemera by incorporating into books some of what I believed relevant and though the original documentation was gone, it was preserved for posterity.[39] However, I was also faced with preserving masses of original documentation that I had gathered over the years which had been given to me with the admonition: 'You will know what to do with these.' To preserve this material, I established archives in appropriate universities and academic institutes.[40]

I was introduced to publishing in 1983 by Tom Turley, the owner of Glendale Press which published the first book I wrote, *Conscience and Conflict: A Biography of Sir Dominic Corrigan, 1802–1880*.[41] The former librarian of the RCPI, Gladys Gardner, had mentioned that papers on Corrigan were entrusted to the College in 1944 by one of his descendants, Francis Cyril Martin. With the help of Gladys's successor, Robert Mills, I found in the basement of the RCPI a trunk of Corrigan's personal and business letters, notebooks, diaries, pamphlets and memorabilia that had lain undisturbed for nearly half a century. This trove of material revealed so many unknown aspects about this remarkable Victorian physician that I was compelled to write his biography.

A Portrait of Irish Medicine: An Illustrated History of Medicine in Ireland was published in 1984 to mark the bicentenary of the RCSI. In this book I wanted to trace the history of Irish medicine through portraiture, sculpture, architecture and other forms of artistic expression in commemorative medals and stained-glass memorials.[42] The project depended on the participation of an art historian with flair and imagination. I found these qualities in the flamboyant personality of Anne Crookshank. Our first meeting was not propitious. On 17 January 1977 on my way home from the hospital, I called on Seán Ó Criadan on Pembroke Road. Ó Criadan had a knowledgable interest in painting and special editions of books.

Shortly after I arrived in Ó Criadan's, Anne Crookshank dropped in, as she often did after leaving Trinity College, where she was Professor of History of Art. Anne's haughty manner and tendency to dismiss those who might steal her limelight didn't appeal to me but this initial assessment was unfounded. Together we visited museums, galleries, medical institutions, churches, cathedrals and private collections, searching for and finding paintings and art that many institutes did not even know they possessed.

Since the book had to make a visual statement, I wanted to produce a de luxe edition with many photographs. Crookshank and I fought over images she wanted for her chapters against those I wanted for mine or other authors. I invariably lost these arguments, but when I look back, Crookshank was right – she was more skilled in curating the images as an assessment of art in medicine. *A Portrait of Irish Medicine* was published, with a limited edition (now sought after by collectors) bearing an embossed spine depicting the early origins of surgeons with the red and white banner of the barber's pole. The book was a tribute to an institution that had survived for two centuries. By articulating her innate appreciation of what was good and what was banal in art, Crookshank directed the reader's attention away from consideration of the curative achievements of doctors and towards their cultural participation in society; she focused on the interaction between science and the humanities in a symbiotic sharing of knowledge, illuminating our understanding of the human condition. As Crookshank said in her opening chapter:

> The doctors of Ireland may congratulate themselves on being the most consistent
> patrons of artists in this country's history. If we had had time to seek out private
> collections more thoroughly, there is no doubt we would have found even more
> medical portraits. But just keeping to the principal public institutions, we have
> seen many hundreds of portraits, oil paintings, sculpture, bronze, stone or marble,
> drawings and miniatures. Many are of high quality, especially in sculpture, where,
> with few exceptions, the main artists working in Ireland are represented by
> excellent work.

In 1984 I felt confident enough to establish my first publishing outlet, the Black Cat Press. During the compilation of *A Portrait of Irish Medicine* I paid frequent visits to Liam Miller, begetter of the Dolmen Press, to learn from this master of book design. Miller designed two books for the Black Cat Press – *Dublin Anatomist: Tom Garry 1884–1963: An Account of the Life of Thomas Peter Garry, Tutor and Prosector in Anatomy, Royal College of Surgeons in Ireland* and the infamous *Dissecting Room Ballads: From the Dublin School of Medicine Fifty Years Ago* by Daragh Smith, or known for short as *Ballads*.

The first edition of *Ballads* has typographical errors, but the explanation for this adds to rather than detracts from the book's provenance. The day shift of male typesetters refused to set obscene literature. The night shift, composed almost exclusively of women, would set it, but the hurried printing schedule didn't allow for proofreading. These typos did not influence laudatory reviews. On 20 September 1985 we held a celebratory dinner in Virginia, County Cavan, to honour Daragh Smith. We presented him with an inscribed copy of *Ballads* and a bronze sculpture by Pat Dolan depicting the last moments of the Sea Baboon. The evening was worthy of recording for posterity, but the cameraman became intoxicated and sent the film to a couple whose wedding he filmed the following day. Some years later the 'Ballads video' finally turned up.[43]

In the 1970s and '80s Dublin experienced an upheaval in hospital care with the closure of many of its voluntary hospitals, some of which had existed for over two centuries. I founded the Anniversary Press to preserve the ethos and esprit de corps in the Charitable Infirmary, the Richmond Hospital and the City of Dublin Skin and Cancer Hospital. I illustrated these historical treatises with photography, believing that imagery often says more than words. Indeed, when I now look at the images of the theatres and wards, at the staff and their dress and modus operandi, I feel vindicated in having captured for future generations the relative simplicity of life, and for illustrating how patients had the comfort of a bed, as distinct from a trolley in a crowded A&E department.

III

6. Literary Dublin

If ever you go to Dublin town
In a hundred years or so …
Patrick Kavanagh, *Collected Poems* (2004)

By the time I qualified as a doctor in 1963, the writers, artists, musicians and freethinkers who created Baggotonia had dispersed owing to emigration, success, failure or death. Yet many of those personalities, though scattered, remained close and introduced me to their literary associates who, in turn, became my friends and often my patients.[1]

Baggotonia stretched from the Grand Canal towards the city along Baggot Street with its meagre flats and studios, past the parks of Fitzwilliam and Merrion to St Stephen's Green and onwards to Grafton Street from which life flowed into side streets on which pubs vied for a clientele that revelled in wit and repartee.[2] Olivia Robertson, a friend of W.B. Yeats, was the first to sense a uniqueness about the area. In the 1950s she wrote:

> Dublin has its own special colony of Bohemia, its 'Latin Quarter', which I shall
> call the 'Baggot Street Quarter'. The Victorian houses are for the most part

transformed into flats; and behind the flats are enticing little lanes with garages. Living over the garages are the artists, whose maisonettes, bravely painted, do indeed remind one of a Chelsea mews.

Newcomers also sensed the energy: 'Ireland wasn't golden always, but it was golden sometimes and in 1950 it was, all in all, a golden age for me and others,' declared Harold Pinter. Brendan Lynch attributed the city's charm to its small size:

> Dublin after the war was a human city. With a population of a little over half a million, a native could leisurely traverse its main streets in half a day, with more than sufficient time to browse, gossip and exchange opinions. Its size and pace encouraged social intercourse; everyone knew everyone. And wit abounded.

The artist Nevill Johnson, originally from England, visited Dublin via Belfast and said: 'The air was bright, and our hearts pumped with the promise of a new world. It seems that at certain epochs men are possessed of a maverick spirit.'[3]

In *Time Pieces; A Dublin Memoir,* John Banville describes Baggotonia as a 'place of magical promise towards which my starved young soul endlessly yearned'. Coming to Dublin from Wexford, he 'settled straight away into the heart of Baggotonia … beyond the borders of which [he] strayed with reluctance'.[4]

The Grand Canal between the locks at Huband Bridge and Baggot Street Bridge was my childhood playground. With my sister and neighbouring children we trod its banks, caught minnows in its shallows and precariously crossed the boards of the locks. Here we often met Patrick Kavanagh, his eyes distorted by the lens of his glasses, talking gruffly to himself, flailing his long arms like sails to propel him onwards or to warm himself on cold days. Thomas Kilroy pictures him stalking 'through the fifties like some *cainteoir* [vagrant satirist] out of the Gaelic past with the sartorial stamp, the swinging coat, the dipped brooding hat, the notorious cough and splutter, arms akimbo, knotted like an embrace that has lost, or crushed its loved object'.[5]

I wonder if my sister and I were among the children Kavanagh had in mind when he wrote the ominous lines:

> On Pembroke Road look out for my ghost
> Dishevelled with shoes untied,
> Playing through the railings with little children
> Whose children have long since died.[6]

When he wasn't patrolling the canal banks, we found him in Parsons Bookshop – where we bought our comics – sitting on a high stool, reading voraciously. It might even be reasonable to assume that he noticed us. As the owner of the bookshop later said: '[Eoin] originally came here as a little boy with his father – whom I remember often warning him not to annoy our resident book advisor of the time, Patrick [Kavanagh].'[7] I remember Kavanagh in Meagher's Chemist where the owner would dispense medication to me according to the prescription my father had given me for one of his patients, and at times I would overhear her patiently dealing with Kavanagh's therapeutic requirements.

As a medical student I lived in Baggotonia. Its characters viewed medical students as their future minders, accepted us as enthusiastic, uncultivated youths who could at least enlighten a conversation with anatomical knowledge should literary testament so demand, or even provide a gratis consultation.

My immersion in the Baggotonian milieu resonates in vignettes and epiphanies of a different age. Sometimes I sit on the bench erected in 1968 by John Ryan and a few loyal friends.[8] The seat, designed by Michael Farrell, is made of oak from County Meath and granite from the Dublin mountains. Inscribed on one side is 'PATRICK KAVANAGH POET 1904–1967, ERECTED BY HIS FRIENDS 17th March 1968' and on the other, 'Lines Written on a Seat on the Grand Canal, Dublin. Erected to the memory of Mrs Dermod O'Brien'. The later bench on the opposite northern bank was unveiled by Mary Robinson in 1991. Sculpted in bronze by John Coll, it depicts Kavanagh with his arms folded and his crumpled hat beside him. While this is a skilfully executed statue of the poet, it fails to capture the atmospheric mood of the original simple bench portrayed by John Ryan in *Remembering How We Stood*:

> In the fullness of summer, when the poplars and beeches crowd the heavens with turbulent foliage, the skies, the trees, and water all seem to merge in one quivering unity. From his seat, you will see the waters of the canal falling 'Niagariously' into the lock, and your vision, as you raise your head, will be led half a mile up the canal until it meets the winking eye of Eustace Bridge. Then, the immense beauty of it all touches the heart. At such a moment one may concede that some parnassian deity (a friend now of the poet) is presiding over the scene.[9]

The canal bank was also visited by Samuel Beckett. When his mother was dying in 1950, he gazed at the nursing-home window overlooking the spot where Kavanagh used to sit, waiting for a sign to tell him his mother's suffering was over – the lowering of the blind, 'one of those dirty brown roller affairs'. Time often draws the threads of existence into proximity in a way that disturbs the random order of life. I learned recently that Kavanagh died in 1967 in the same nursing-home room overlooking the canal.[10]

Sitting on the Kavanagh bench I often wonder how fearful it must have been for him when his life was threatened there. The attempted murder is a topic of fascination in biographical works on the poet.[11] David Davison's contemporaneous account of the event is particularly intriguing. David was a trainee photographer in The Green Studio Ltd, owned by Reggie Wiltshire and his wife, Elinor, who knew Kavanagh. David writes:

One morning … the Wiltshires were uncharacteristically late … In the early hours of the morning, they had been awoken by knocking on the door and found Paddy standing there in a most dishevelled muddy condition. It transpired that a vicious Dublin gang was furious with him because as a contributor to *The Irish Farmers Journal* he had exposed one of their profitable rackets. At that time Irish farmers were installing proper steel field gates as replacements for the less secure Heath-Robinson structures commonly found around the country at that time. These replacements were generally of a high quality but the gang in question had sourced much inferior products of similar appearance and were actively selling them as the superior article. Paddy's exposé threatened this racket and they wanted revenge. Subsequently two gang members sought him out in his favourite pub and while behaving in a friendly manner slipped something into his drink. He soon appeared to be staggering on his feet, not so unusual in his case, his two 'friends' volunteered to help him home and taking a firm hold set off from the pub. However, instead of heading home they made their way to the Grand Canal and having reached a nearby bridge they tossed Paddy over the parapet and quickly made their escape, knowing that it was plausible for a drunken man to fall into the canal and drown with no suspicion falling on them. Over the years young fellows up to no good have found it amusing to open sluice gates on the canal locks and drain sections down to a small trickle. Fortunately for Kavanagh this had been done to the stretch into which he was dumped, and his fall had been broken by landing in soft mud. Some hours later he came to, crawled out and made his way to the Wiltshires' flat … He then returned to the same pub and gained some satisfaction from the shocked expressions on the culprits' faces.

Many of Kavanagh's fellow writers have commented on how he secured this part of Dublin as his terrain. Benedict Kiely suggests that his new-found territory 'needed to make him think he was walking up and down the main street of Carrickmacross on a market day'. Anthony Cronin claimed that it became a substitute for his homeland village:

> This was his village. It contained what he would have regarded as the necessities of life – three or four pubs, a couple of bookmakers and a bookshop. And he patrolled this area, he knew everything about its life, he knew all the people in its pubs, all the gin-drinking land-ladies in The Waterloo lounge, all the Baggot Street irregulars, all the soaks, all the girls who were in digs round there he'd stop them in the streets and ask them questions about their progress in exams or their boyfriends or their jobs. There can hardly ever have been an area of a city so intensively patrolled.[12]

Niall Sheridan, who knew Kavanagh well, delighted in his verbal tirades. Kavanagh conducted his ever-troubled financial affairs in a bank at the corner of Harry Street and Grafton Street, managed by a Mr Colthurst. Niall recalled seeing Kavanagh emerging from the bank with Colthurst en route to McDaid's and it was evident from the thunder on Kavanagh's face that things hadn't gone well. This was confirmed when Kavanagh shouted for all to hear: 'Colthurst, you are a shit of the vilest hue', to which the bank manager, unperturbed, replied: 'Kavanagh, flattery will not advance your cause one whit.'

As with Kavanagh, my recollections of Brendan Behan date back to childhood, but, unlike Kavanagh, we kept our distance from Behan – his behaviour could be unpredictable. I came to know him more intimately during my studentship and as a young doctor in the late 1950s. I preferred to avoid him when he was in a mood of drunken offensiveness, but there were moments when the kindness of his character shone through the dark cloud of alcoholism that dominated his life. When we met, he always addressed me as 'Doc' and I would only call him Brendan when we were in the convivial ambience of McDaid's.

One night in McDaid's I witnessed a rare occurrence with Behan and Kavanagh (who were rarely civil to each other, Behan having dubbed Kavanagh as 'the fucker from Mucker' and 'Paddy the wanker') clasping each other arm in arm with a pint in their free hands, tottering on a table, singing 'The Sash My Father Wore'. All was going well until Behan crashed to the floor. As he surfaced, shouting expletives at the assembly, pandemonium erupted before the establishment returned to 'normality' and conversation resumed as though nothing had happened.

Sometimes, after McDaid's closed, the well-oiled assembly would wend its way to a notorious venue called the Catacombs in the basement of 13 Fitzwilliam Place, where drunken conversation continued until dawn. Tony Cronin, who lived above the Catacombs, described how the empty bottles were redeemed the following day for cash by the landlord, Dickie Wyman. I went to the Catacombs in my first year in medicine with an older student, Jack McDonagh. We were checked at the entrance, and, having the passport of a brown bag of bottles, we were admitted to a dimly lit room with a central dais on which someone was warbling a song. We sat on cushions drinking and talking, when there was hush and a figure with a grand accent announced that there would shortly be an 'execution'. This was greeted with applause but McDonagh led me to exit and warned me: 'Get the hell out of this place as fast as you can.' I fled, not knowing if McDonagh considered the 'execution' too shocking for my tender years or if I was to be the victim of the event. Behan captured the decadence of this retreat of iniquity: 'There was some sort of a party practically every night at the Catacombs. A crowd of people would assemble in the flat, each bringing a bottle of gin, or whiskey, or a dozen of stout. There would be men having women, men having men and women having women; a fair field and no favour.'[13]

Apart from meeting Behan in McDaid's, I only had two intimate encounters with him, notable for dispelling the popular image of a drunken debauchee hurtling invective at all and sundry. These meetings left me with a regard for his generosity and ease of expression. Once, Kevin Duffy and I went to Toners in Baggot Street, and as we sipped our pints, an unmistakable voice boomed: 'Is that a fucking Manchester University scarf around youse neck?' I replied it was from a girl I met when I was working in a Manchester brewery during the summer. On foot of this, Behan invited us to join him, and hearing that we were impecunious medical students, the drinks thereafter – and there were many – were on him.

He had pleasant memories of Manchester, where he had befriended 'dear Joan Littlewood'. He discussed the curse of the gentry whose presence besmirched the island, declaring an Anglo-Irish gentleman to be a 'bollocks on a horse'. He recalled with pleasure how he had visited the house of one such, whose ancestors had been granted 400 acres of land – when the tide was out. Most enduring was his pride in knowing where he had been conceived: 'Any idiot knows where he was born, but I know where I was fucking well conceived.' The event occurred – his mother had shown him the exact spot – 'under a tree in Stephen's Green, on a summer's evening'. Nine months before his birthday, he would visit the tree and bow down to it. Onlookers would remark upon his behaviour, not knowing he was paying homage to his place of conception.

My next brief meeting with Behan was in the Richmond Hospital where I was working as a house physician. He had been admitted for diabetes, and some days after his discharge, I met him wandering in the hall of the doctors' residence with a package under his arm. I asked if I could help, and he said he had a small gift for the Polish lady doctor who had been kind to him. It was a signed copy of *The Borstal Boy*. Not many patients go to such lengths to thank their doctors.

When Sylvia Beach visited Dublin, she wanted to meet Behan, so Niall Sheridan arranged this at his house in Monkstown, where Beach was staying. Behan, accompanied by his wife, Beatrice, arrived sober and impeccably dressed. Niall exclaimed: 'He looked like a bank manager.' The evening passed uneventfully in pleasant conversation, at the end of which Beach remarked to Niall: 'I wonder if his publicity is greater than his talent.'

At a party hosted by Niall and his wife, Monica, John Ryan recounted how 'an awful American lady, with a blue rinse' sidled up to Behan and asked the question all writers abhor: 'What is the message in your writing?' Behan replied: 'Madam, if I wish to send messages, I use the Trans-American Express.' This led Niall to wallow in the humour of Behan's dictum on the distinction between prose and poetry. How easily the poorly rhyming words

> There was a young fella named Rollocks,
> Who worked for Ferrier Pollocks,
> As he walked on the strand
> With a girl by the hand,
> The water came up to his … ankles.

could have been transformed into poetry had the tide been in.

I once suggested to Ulick O'Connor that his biography of Oliver St John Gogarty was his best book, but O'Connor was more interested in discussing his biography of Behan, written in 1970. Most critics decried the book because O'Connor had referred to Behan's homosexual tendencies. John Ryan dismissed the matter as irrelevant, saying: 'Brendan would have mounted a Drimnagh bus if the urge was on him.' Denis Johnston, never one to mince his words, brought the conversation to a terse end with: 'But, Ulick, it is not a good book!'

Like Kavanagh and Behan, Micheál Mac Liammóir was an ever-present figure in my youth. I even remember accompanying my father on a doctor's visit to his house on Harcourt Terrace. I also recall my parents discussing in hushed tones the homosexual relationship between Mac Liammóir and Hilton Edwards, which was known throughout Dublin and was accepted, albeit with a humorous comment that was not always genteel. Once, when Edwards and Mac Liammóir were entertaining at home, the actor Paddy Bedford arrived, in his cups, declaring: 'Jaysus, Micheál, the jacks, where's the effing jacks?' to which Mac Liammóir replied, 'Proceed, my good man, to the end of the hall where you will see a door with the sign "Gentlemen", but let this not deter you for a moment and proceed straight in.'

I first saw Mac Liammóir acting in his one-man shows of immense beauty and strength, *The Importance of Being Oscar*, in 1960, which was followed by *I Must Be Talking to My Friends* in 1963, and I had enjoyed the memoir of his theatrical life, *All for Hecuba*. I welcomed the opportunity of a chance meeting, which happened in 1976 when Tona and I were on the ferry from Rosslare to Le Havre. I was in a queue at a hatch from which a sullen girl served a murky coffee when my spirits were lifted on hearing the unmistakable rich voice proclaim: 'Hilton, do you mean to say that they are unable to separate the milk from the tea on this damnable tub?' And there, standing with a dripping paper cup, was Mac Liammóir, out of place in the grim cafeteria. He was placated eventually by Hilton, who left him sitting at a small table smoking and gazing wistfully towards the sea. I introduced myself, and, when I recalled my father's visit to his house in my childhood, he welcomed me to his table. He discussed his childhood, his early acting career, Noel Coward and Colette, whom he 'adored':

> Oh, how I would love to have met her. She was, of course, old when she died, in her eighties, I think. The world waited for Jean Cocteau, her great friend, to speak and satisfy its morbid curiosity about Colette. But he was so shaken, so upset, and so honourable, and he was, as you know, queer, and she, the darling, was everything – that all he could say was: 'We loved as brother and sister, as man and woman, she was my dearest friend.' Don't you think that is beautiful, truly beautiful?[14]

When I met Mac Liammóir weeks later and asked how he had enjoyed Tours after the awful trip from Rosslare, he said he'd had a wonderful time because he had made a new friend. This friend had become a Buddhist 'to his own great happiness and to the utter misery of all his friends. And so there he was, my dear boy, sublime in spiritual ecstasy with all his dear friends in the doldrums. Very selfish of him, don't you think?' Niall Sheridan, on hearing this egocentric declaration, remarked: 'Surely the greatest happiness one can hope for is to see one's friends in misery on one's own behalf.'

My most poignant memory of Mac Liammóir was in 1977 when Denis Johnston asked if I would accompany him and Mac Liammóir to the revival of *The Old Lady Says 'No'!* in the Abbey. I collected Johnston and we met Mac Liammóir and a friend at the theatre and went straight to our seats. The production was bad. Mac Liammóir and Johnston knew it. The only light relief was when Robert Emmet asked: 'Is there a doctor in the house?' and Johnston murmured to me: 'Now's your chance, Eoin.'

Sadness overcame me during the performance. I tried to fathom Mac Liammóir's feelings a half-century after the first production when, by all accounts, he was outstanding as Robert Emmet. Had the direction of Edwards and the acting of Mac Liammóir given the first production its magic? After the performance, Mac Liammóir went to the bar but Johnston, who was not in a talkative mood, remained in his seat. When the audience dispersed, we left quietly.

Although Nevill Johnson was an active artistic force in Baggotonia, I didn't meet him until the 1980s when he was exhibiting at Tom Caldwell's gallery. We established a bond of humour, a *joie de vivre*, and shared the view that artistic endeavour was a means of 'cheating the gods' by leaving a statement, however small, that would endure as a declaration of having existed. Nevill gave me his autobiography, *The Other Side of Six*, which portrays a sensitive, rebellious intellectual confronting a conventional and privileged upbringing in favour of a life devoted to artistic expression through painting.[15]

When Nevill left England for Belfast he met John Luke, who taught him to paint. The pair became close friends, even though Nevill regarded Luke as too accomplished a draughtsman to be a good painter. In Northern Ireland, Nevill had to reconcile the dichotomy of viewing the horrors of World War II from the safety of a faraway pinnacle while being beset with guilt, which, if not to be expiated, was alleviated by painting. His unhappiness deepened when his wife became 'enamoured of a rising young painter from Dublin.'[16] In 1949 'a lone and rather bewildered man of thirty-eight' entered Baggotonia where he, like Kavanagh and so many others, paused at the bridge on the Grand Canal to enjoy the 'washed grass and fresh watered elms'. Thus refreshed, he found lodgings on Raglan Road and established himself as one of the most significant artistic figures in the Baggotonian movement, to which he bequeathed a rich legacy of painting and photography.

In Dublin, Nevill met the art dealer Victor Waddington, who, by providing him with modest financial security, enabled him to paint. In 1952 he obtained a grant from the Arts Council with which he purchased a second-hand Leica and, accompanied by the ever-loyal Anne Yeats,[17] immersed himself in the Liberties, where he became a trusted figure among the habitués of that impoverished part of the city. His photographs exude a wonderful pathos, capturing the warmth of personality in the portraits of slum tenants, joxers on the dole, workers on bicycles or tending their horses, dockers, clergy, the down-and-outs and the occupants of the lowly pubs downing the elixir of momentary peace and forgetfulness. These unique images portray a city and its people poised to step from an aeonian past into a turbulent future.[18]

Consideration was given to producing a film documentary on Nevill's Dublin photographs but funding didn't become available. This correspondence illustrates Nevill's sceptical view of so-called progress and development in Dublin:

> The giantism of a cathedral carries its own logic: the awe we feel is generated for a purpose and is expected. But the gross brutality of many buildings of today exhibits a fearful insensitivity, many of them bearing all the 'earmarks of an eyesore', as the man said. We humans are dwarfed, bullied and chivvied around by these monstrous structures, our stature denied, our pride ignored. And there are to be found no idiosyncratic corners for our surprise.

Nevill also deplored the destruction of community:

> I suppose that in the name of growth and progress we must accept impersonal supermarkets and the din of traffic. So, it's goodbye to the corner shop and goodbye to the slums of Gardiner Street; life there was certainly coarse, risky and ungracious. But surely the isolation of suburban estates breeds its own insults and despair.

The art critic Dickon Hall stressed how much Dublin is in Nevill's debt: 'His legacy to Ireland is a collection of paintings and photographs that examine, criticise, explore and celebrate its landscape and its cities, its culture, industries and society, in a manner that no other artist of the time achieved.'[19]

But even Dublin couldn't hold Nevill indefinitely. He moved to Chalk Farm in London where Cedra Castellain, 'a notably beautiful woman', gave him shelter with painters Robert Colquhoun and Robert MacBryde. He married Margaret

Pettigrew and inherited money with which he acquired the right and title to four cottages at Wilby Green, near Framlingham in Suffolk. During this period he kept a diary which, unlike *The Other Side of Six*, is a private chronicle giving us insight into the mind of the artist grappling with the creative process.

My medical research brought me to London frequently, and I was able to meet Nevill often. We'd met in the Churchill Arms on Kensington Church Street and discuss literature, life, politics, his past, his painting and how best to propagate his work. We also discussed science, which he believed could abolish the myths of expression and reference; he regarded scientists as 'the most revolutionary and iconoclastic of men'. In one of our discussions on reductionism in art, Nevill surprised me by asserting that colour would have to be removed from imagery, which he equated as equivalent to 'getting God out of one's life'. I agreed with this concept for photographic art, perhaps, but for painting, I wasn't so sure. 'There will come a time,' he said, 'when colour will be unfashionable – colour is rather feminine – nothing wrong with that, but the day of the "colourist" will pass, as has the day of God.'

One day Nevill invited me back to his spartan flat in Peel Street, which served as a studio, 'to share the mood he was transmitting to canvas'. He showed me ten or so canvases that astounded me. I asked if he had suffered in their execution. He asked why I thought there might have been pain. I told him I sensed in the paintings a personal intensity that had culminated in an Augustinian catharsis on canvas. Nevill admitted that the creation of a painting could invoke pain but the painting was only successful if it imparted the suffering of the creative process to the beholder. Apart from the autobiographical release I saw in these paintings, I identified a quality I also sensed in Beckett's writing:

> Much of the apparently surrealistic in Beckett's writing is linked, sometimes very positively, sometimes only tenuously, with the reality of existence, and much of this existence emanates from memories of Dublin, a world rendered almost unrecognisable by Beckett's technique of denuding his landscape and its people (while also annihilating time) in his creation of the 'unreality of the real'.[20]

Was Nevill not expressing similar sentiments when he wrote:

> I spy psychiatrists and neurologists waiting in the wings. Let them come to the podium and state their case … I'm not denying the role of intellect; with it we can build a frame on which to pin our claims. Then, if the song rings true, we can kick away the props and it will stand.

The paintings in Peel Street achieved what he and Beckett aspired to: he had kicked the props to hell and the edifice was left, resplendent in its sturdiness.

During my visits to Peel Street, I tried to help Nevill overcome doubt by restoring his confidence, urging him to keep painting, not to compromise, and to allow the 'mood of the moment' to influence his brush. On one of my visits, some of the paintings were gone. Knowing that he no longer sold his paintings, I asked what happened to a painting I had admired on an earlier visit. He replied, 'Eoin, I devour my children.' Now my visits became missions of mercy with the purpose of saving as many of the 'children' as I could – some thirty or so – by taking them back to Dublin for framing. In 1995 Nevill attended an exhibition of his work at the Solomon Gallery in Dublin, which unfortunately was not well attended.[21]

I was increasingly intrigued by Nevill's writings. I recognized three artistic personae struggling for expression where painting and photography took precedence over writing. So, when he asked me in May 1999 to be his literary executor, I set about publishing his writings. In the 1980s neither of us could have anticipated that thirty years later we would toil over the proofs of *The Other Side of Six* for a revised edition. During meetings he was evasive about the mysterious title, preferring to leave it uninterpreted. Recently, I unearthed a short story he wrote bearing the same title. The protagonist is a physicist and a 'maverick thorn in the flesh of academic scholars … for his penetrating attacks on formal and mathematical logic'. He propounds his development of an enantiomorphic faculty, which, by providing him with a mirror image of his mind, allows him entry to a world where 'time is quantized and non-lineal – in short, "the other side of six". This takes us closer to meaning, which nonetheless remains obscure'.

I also prepared *Tractatus Pudicus* for publication in which Nevill gives a poetic rendering of Dublin life and decadence:

I wish to speak of Dublin in the
fifties, the last decade of domination
by the Church and the Nation
myth.

To speak of Convent Place and the young
opera singer sitting naked in her
fur coat.

Of Count Taafe [*sic*] and the emeralds
of Ruth Latif the spangled belly
dancer.

The last decade of Nevill's life was preoccupied with ill health: 'On shaky legs I entered the winter of my seventieth year, a sad bag of muscle and gut, humbled and prepared to listen. "Take it easy," they said, "and you'll last a few years yet."' He lasted quite a few years longer, painted continuously and, true to form, destroyed much of his work. I helped orchestrate his medical treatment with specialists. He considered the prospect of death: 'Death had been up till now something in the papers, something in a little parlour in Belfast – my mother suffered not so much death as a kind of weariness; she turned off the light, handed in the counterfoil. But now I saw death manifest in the street; it stood at the bus stop, sat in the pub.' On my last meeting with him in the Middlesex Hospital, he looked from me standing at his bed to the catheter draining him like an hourglass that would never be inverted, and with eyes of sadness, sadness in the realization that his time had passed and mine not quite so, we parted on a quote from the second Book of Samuel: 'How are the mighty fallen, and the weapons of war perished!'

I am grateful to Nevill for the enrichment he brought to my life. I promised him that I would do what I could to bring his work to wider attention. I arranged exhibitions, edited publications and established an archive and scholarship in UCD to facilitate access to this polymath's works and to enable future scholarship. Despite these endeavours, Nevill remains largely unappreciated. His paintings excite little interest at international auctions, his photographic archive doesn't receive the critical acclaim it merits and his writings have not received scholarly attention. But, as is so often the case when genius is in our midst, we fail to appreciate its presence. The time will come when Nevill will be recognized as an influential twentieth-century intellectual who, apart from mastering the art of surrealistic painting, explored the philosophy of expression and the relationship of art to the vagaries of human existence:

> A young man with a water colour sketch
> Turns his head, his eyes serious, deferential
> 'Sir, could you advise me'
> 'Yes, boy, put a bag over your head and paint the smell of grass.'

I met Niall Sheridan in Eugene and Mai Lambert's house in the 1970s.[22] Eugene entertained in the pillared room of his house overlooking the sea where conversation flowed as liberally as the wine, with Mai lavishing cuisine on the company, which included writers, actors, producers and TV personalities. After that, Niall and I often met in our homes or local hostelries, such as Goggin's, and restaurants around the city. He became a dear friend, and I appreciated his unique genius and dissipated talent.[23] He was a raconteur par excellence, and good raconteurs, like actors, must hold the attention of the audience which may necessitate interpreting the truth liberally.

I tried to persuade Niall to write a memoir. He said 'that once the ink started flowing the book would take on its own structure'. We agreed that this *recherche du temps perdu* should be 'cloaked in the mists of nostalgia and that a chronological sequence was not desirable'. Furthermore, 'out of respect for O'Nolan and Joyce, the book should have neither a beginning nor an end or be restricted by the convention of chapters and the like'. However, when he admitted that he would be satisfied to 'die happily, having been privileged not only to know so many interesting and talented people but to have been their trusted contemporaries', I realized that he would not conform to the discipline of committing his past to paper.

Niall's childhood was filled with sadness. His father was a complex person, 'a most noble man'. He had been well-to-do with 500 acres of land, but being idealistic and principled, he lost it in pursuing his vision for a 'new Ireland'. Among his achievements was the publication of the paper *Sinn Féin* in Oldcastle, County Meath. He later gave Arthur Griffith permission to use the name for his political party. He was imprisoned for his political activities when Niall was young, so he became the 'surrogate patriarch' of the household.

Niall described his mother as 'a soft lady' whose gentle life in Northern Ireland 'fitted her for little other than running up accounts in drapery stores'. However, when left with a family to rear and a husband's cause to fight, 'strange to behold she showed her mettle'. IRA members were often given shelter in the household, and one of Niall's boyhood tasks was to carry guns to the old dairy close to a neighbour's house so weapons were hidden from unwelcome visitors. The Black and Tans, aware of the political leanings of the Sheridan family, were regular and unwelcome visitors. A childhood event haunted Niall. He discussed it with me only twice when we were alone and had had a few drinks. One evening a drunken Black and Tan plucked Niall's fifteen-month-old brother from his mother's arms and flung the infant to the fireplace, cracking his skull and killing him instantly. I think it did Niall good to discuss this event that caused him deep anguish, but he wasn't bitter, preferring to 'adopt my father's philosophy, which was that bitterness hurts oneself more than the object of that sentiment'.

When he was very young, Niall's nearest national school was five miles away so he was educated by an aunt who was fluent in French and a Latin scholar. When he was sent the national school for the first time at the age of eleven he felt out of place. He excelled in languages but was relegated to the 'baby' class for maths. He was next educated by the Marist Fathers in Dundalk where he earned a scholarship for UCD.

I often questioned Niall about his literary friends. Charlie Donnelly, whose poetry I admired, had been the subject of a recent television documentary, *Even the Olives Are Bleeding*, which had brought his life into focus. Niall, his contemporary at UCD, regarded him as one of the most mature minds he'd ever encountered. He was saddened by his death in the Spanish Civil War and regretted that the futility of idealism had robbed Ireland of one of its brightest literary minds.

When I admired *Twenty Poems*, which Niall had written jointly with Donagh McDonagh in 1934, he dismissed the praise: 'Eoin, when you are faced with the poetry of WBY, poetic ambition falters before the work of such genius.' We also discussed Denis Devlin's *The Heavenly Foreigner*, for which he had written the foreword. Niall had been fond of Devlin, who died from cancer in St Vincent's Hospital in 1959. He had asked to see Niall hours before his death but passed away before Niall arrived – his failure to be with his friend in his hour of need caused him deep regret.

Another poet, Austin Clarke, according to Niall, feared heights, which he overcame in his dotage when he took to air flight, having previously been terrified in a lift. To finance these globetrotting forays, he recast his earlier poems (published in forgotten journals and newspapers) using an old-fashioned typewriter and sold the manuscripts to an American university. Seamus Heaney, with whom Niall's wife, Monica, was friendly and to whom Heaney had dedicated a poem, was, in Niall's opinion, the best living poet in Ireland. Monica's wit was such that Niall turned the aphorism she had once applied to Niall Montgomery by asserting *sotto voce* that she could 'clip a hedge with her tongue'.[24] Monica was utterly unpredictable and likely to shock even the most liberal souls. Her unpredictability was so reliable that Niall once remarked: 'I cannot stand creatures of habit – come to think of it, Monica's unpredictability is becoming a habit – I must talk to her!'

Niall was an authority on horse racing, having been racing correspondent for *The Irish Field*. He was a gambler and dissipated much of the family's meagre funds on sorties to the bookmakers. People saw him as 'a bit of a paradox' as he walked around the parade ring with Eliot's *The Waste Land* protruding from one

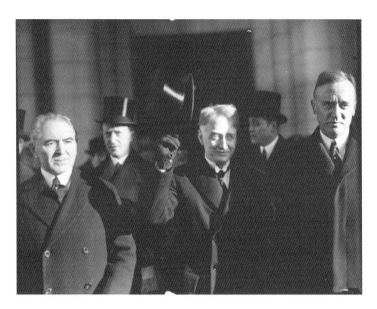

President W.T. Cosgrave (centre) with Ambassador Timothy Smiddy (left) and William Castle Jr, Assistant Secretary of State, being cheered on arrival in Washington in 1928. Desmond FitzGerald is behind, on the left. Courtesy of Colum Kenny.

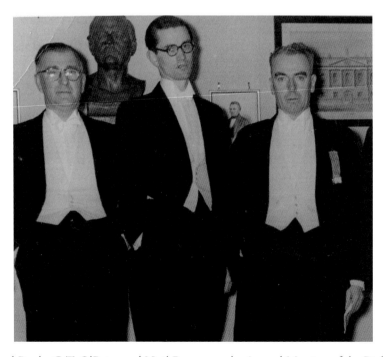

Michael Brady, G.T. O'Brien and Noël Browne at the Annual Meeting of the Biological Society of the Royal College of Surgeons in Ireland in 1948. Private collection.

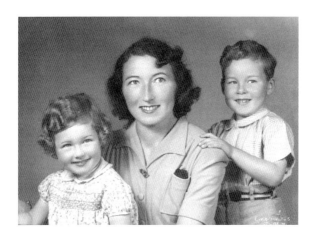

Muriel O'Brien with her son, Eoin, and daughter, Berna, 1944. Private collection.

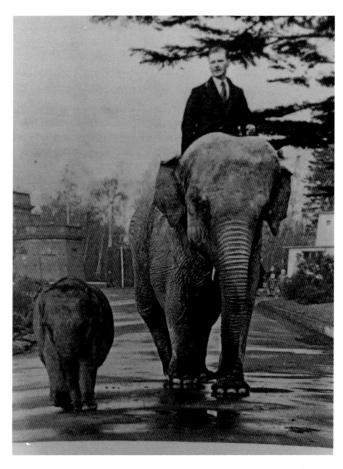

Jim Kenny, the elephant keeper, astride Sarah and accompanied by Komali, c. 1940.
Courtesy of Paul and Pat Kenny.

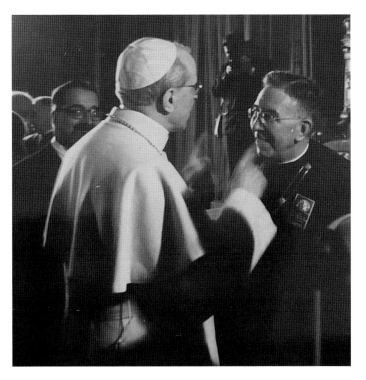

Pope Pius XII being updated on astronomical issues by Daniel O'Connell, c. 1950.
Courtesy of Geraldine O'Brien.

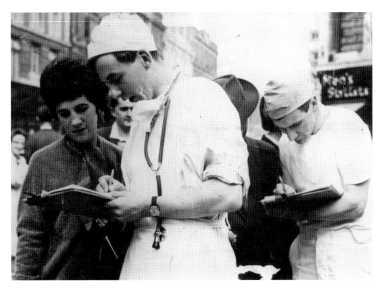

Eoin O'Brien and Tom McDonald collecting names for a charitable petition on
O'Connell Street, 1963. Private collection.

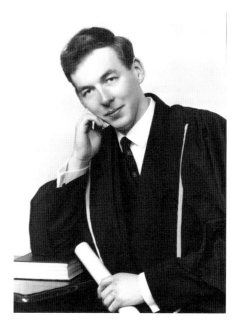

Graduation photograph of Eoin O'Brien, 1963. Private collection.

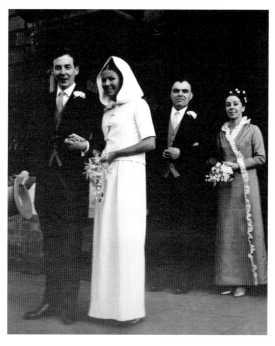

Eoin and Tona O'Brien on their wedding day, 27 May 1968, at Newman University
Church with Pat Rafferty and Maura Lee. Private collection.

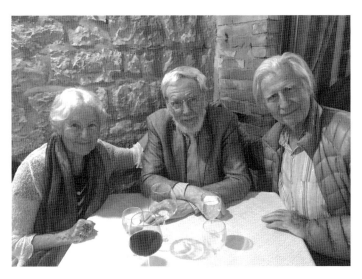

Eoin O'Brien with Brian and Barbara O'Doherty at Todi, Italy, 2015. Private collection.

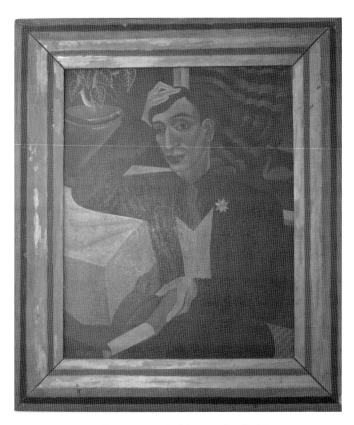

Portrait of Con Leventhal by Cecil Salkeld, 2022.
Courtesy of Peter and Andrew Woolfson.

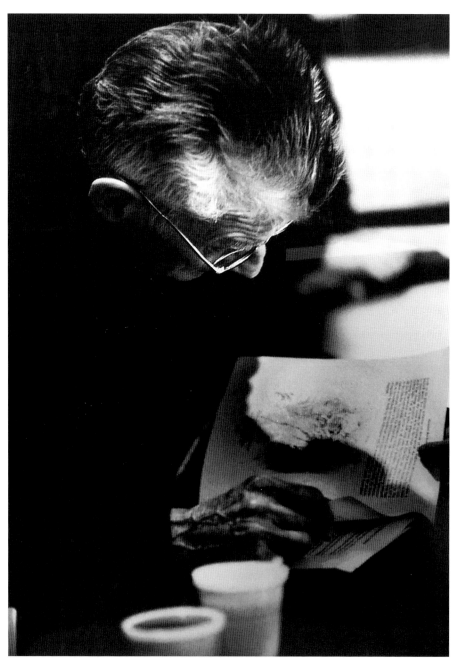

Samuel Beckett in 1984 studying his portrait by Avigdor Arikha in
A.J. Leventhal, 1896–1979: Dublin Scholar, Wit and Man of Letters, edited by
Eoin O'Brien. Courtesy of John Minihan.

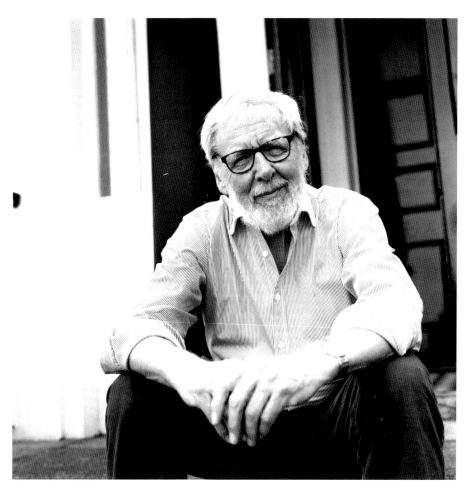

Eoin O'Brien at his Dublin home, 2017. Courtesy of John Minihan.

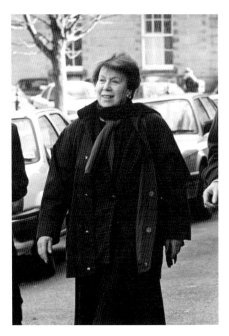

Barbara Bray at the presentation of her correspondence to the Library of Trinity College Dublin, 13 February 1997. Courtesy of Jane Maxwell, Library of Trinity College Dublin.

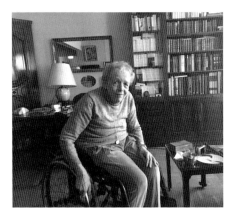

Edith Fournier, 2017. Courtesy of Eoin O'Brien.

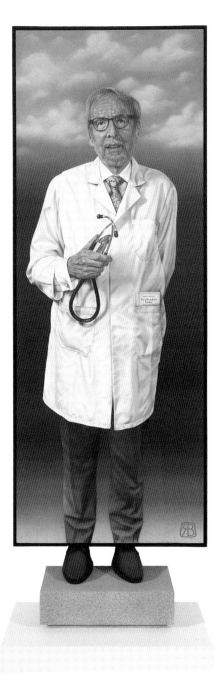

Portrait of Eoin O'Brien by Robert Ballagh, 2022. Courtesy of The Charles Institute, University College Dublin.

pocket and *Timeform* from the other. One of the racing characters remembered by Niall was 'the Pisser Bourke', 'a sort of henchman and runner to the trainer More O'Ferrall'. According to Niall, O'Ferrall's avarice was relentless in this period of decline in Count John McCormack's career. The Pisser asked O'Ferrall if they should not support their patron, who was singing in the Theatre Royal, to which he replied: 'Singing in the Royal! When we're finished with him, he'll be singing outside the place.'

The Toucher Doyle was another racing acquaintance of Niall's. Such was his amiability and wit, he gained entry to the most expensive enclosures at race meetings in England by staying close to racegoers of eminence. On one occasion, when sidling into the members' enclosure at Aintree Racecourse on the tails of W.J. Kelly (proprietor of a well-known tailors in Grafton Street), he was stopped by the door steward: 'I say, and where do you think you're going?' The Toucher claimed he was a member of Mr Kelly's entourage, to which the steward replied, 'We 'ave the governor, we 'ave the trainer, the first groom, the stable lad, so who the hell do you think you are?' to which the Toucher responded: 'Well then, I can only be the fucking horse!'

Another racing vignette concerned a reverend priest named Healy from Bray who, boarding the train for Dublin, joined the carriage of three bookmakers bound for Aintree via the North Wall and Liverpool. Needing a fourth member for a game of poker, the reverend was invited to join them, but he declined, saying 'I never play poker for three reasons. Firstly, I do not have any money and …' when he was interrupted by one of the bookmakers with, 'And you can stick the other two [reasons] up your arse!'

In return for medical care, Niall presented me with a tape of James Joyce reading Anna Livia Plurabelle, with the dedication 'To Eoin, who knows what it is all about.' The recording was chilling – it was as though another presence had entered the room. It is a symphony in words – beautiful music, neither poetry nor prose but a unique blending of speech and composition by a master of literary innovation. It set me wondering if one did not have to be a Dubliner to fully appreciate *Finnegans Wake*?

Through Niall I met the composer Malcolm Arnold who moved to Dublin in the 1970s to escape domestic difficulties in England. He befriended the Sheridans, who introduced him to the Dublin literati. Arnold was a man of exquisite manners; even when inebriated, he exuded charm.[25] During his time in Dublin we met often and went to many restaurants where he enjoyed testing their epicurean capabilities. Arnold was enraptured with the city and its inhabitants but unfortunately the pub ambience aggravated his alcoholism, which was sad to witness.

At one stage Arnold had difficulty passing urine, so I arranged for him to be admitted to Monkstown Hospital, where my colleague David Lane, apart from being an accomplished musician, was deft with the scalpel. Lane confirmed that circumcision was necessary, which, although it was a trivial procedure, did not stop Arnold from recuperating in the hospital. Here, he settled into the care of the nurses, holding court, receiving visitors and discussing life with the liberality of thought that follows the imbibement of a carefully chosen claret. We discussed what should be done with the foreskin remnant. Tona suggested a purse, or was she doing him an injustice – perhaps a portmanteau? Niall declared the occasion too great to pass into oblivion. Standing at the foot of Arnold's bed, he read a panegyric to mark the maestro's deliverance:

> Now that the surgeon's work is finished,
> Must Malcolm play a fifth diminished?
> No! Mighty monarch of the trumpet,
> Full many a tired but happy strumpet,
> Awakening, blear-eyed in the morn,
> Recalls that monumental horn.
> Not Giscard, Kissinger or Heath
> Could such a noble sword unsheath,
> And leave behind a relic slight,
> But subject to full copyright.
>
> And so, dear friends, be not afraid
> At hidden treasure now displayed;
> No need to worry any further
> When Priapus comes out of purdah;
> No need to tremble or beware
> The fate of Sampson minus hair.
> Fear no diminuendo. Mark,
> He's kept the trunk but shed the bark.
> And with this happy thought I close;
> It's no skin off the Maestro's nose!

Arnold vowed to set it to music with a brass band and full chorus in the Cardiff Arms Park. Likewise, when Niall gave Arnold a copy of Brian O'Nolan's

At Swim-Two-Birds, he resolved to compose a musical tribute to the work. Furthermore, he determined to moderate his consumption of alcohol by henceforth drinking only 'pints of plain'.

However, this didn't last for long. One evening in Goggin's, after many 'pints of plain', Arnold admitted he missed a good claret. He went on to discuss the vintage of wines, which led, as often happens in pub banter, to a far-removed topic. Arnold recalled Sir John Barbirolli conducting a rehearsal when the awfulness of one viola player prompted him to ask: 'What year did you leave the Academy?' The unfortunate player replied, 'Nineteen-forty-seven.' Barbirolli muttered, 'Oh dear, a very bad year for violas.' After the pub closed, Arnold and I went to my home on Clifton Terrace, where we drank a tad too much wine. The recordings we played attest to our increasing inebriation – Kodály's folk music, the *Missa Luba*, Verdi's *Requiem*, Richard Harris singing *MacArthur Park* and Jack MacGowran speaking Beckett. We discussed Arnold's life, his broken marriages, his love of children, and his love for Tona, 'the most beautiful woman I have ever met'.

Niall is portrayed as Brinsley in O'Nolan's *At Swim-Two-Birds* and he often recounted his visit to Joyce in Paris, to whom he had brought a copy of the novel, a bottle of Jameson, and Hafner's sausages, all of which greatly pleased Joyce.

My daughter, Aphria, who could not resist leaving her bed to eavesdrop on parties, was seen by Niall as deserving of commemoration, and he wrote 'The Night Watch', on her second birthday on 2 April 1978:

You go to bed so early
And, oh, so quietly.
You never stir till dawn comes up
Across the Irish Sea.
Well, perhaps a fleeting visit,
Just to see what's going on
(You can always tell your mother
You were going to the John).
Then a second short safari,
A toddle down the stairs,
Keeps one so well informed
On the state of world affairs.
Next time (Ha! Ha! Hey Presto!)
You appear out of the air.
Of course you aren't spying –

You just *happen* to be there.
Soon you'll fix the silly adults,
Who keep sending you away,
For one of these fine evenings,
You'll toddle down – and STAY.

Another inducement for Niall's mischievous humour arose when I told him about my grandfather Audo Smiddy's affair with Mrs Agnes McFeat during his time as Minister Plenipotentiary in Washington. Niall set about composing a limerick:

The bilingual Mrs McFeat
Moved smoothly among the elite
But went churlish and giddy
When caressed by Smiddy
As she sighed: 'Je viens, mais trop vite.'

The letter accompanying the limerick closed with: 'The line in French celebrates, of course, a physiological event not necessarily connected with actual movement within our time-space continuum. Yours in the odour of sanctity, Niall.'

I attempted to write poetry and discussed poetic structure with Niall, an example being Gogarty's 'The Image-Maker', which we regarded as magnificent (almost as perfect as Philip Larkin's 'Cut Grass'). It made us wonder if W.B. Yeats might not have been right in dubbing him the greatest lyric poet of the age.

Niall was so fascinated by Gogarty that I arranged for him to address the RCSI students in 1975. He received a standing ovation after sharing his reminiscences of the man, which concluded with his verse 'On a Fallen Electrician'.[26] Two large electrical signs marred Dublin's skyline in the 1930s: one for BOVRIL in College Green cast its iridescent message towards Westmoreland Street and O'Connell Street; the other, for OXO, commanded the attention of the denizens of Nassau Street. The latter was situated on a tall building beside Fanning's Pub – now the Lincoln Inn, then owned by Senator Fanning. One day the first O in OXO failed to light, and an electrician named Joe, known not only for his professional prowess but for his wit and geniality, was summoned to fix it. But having dallied in Fanning's beforehand, he slipped from the rooftop to his death on the pavement below. That evening there was an air of gloom in Fanning's, where Brinsley McNamara, Austin Clarke, Fred Higgins and Seumas O'Sullivan were among the gathering. Oliver St John Gogarty joined the company, and the bartending senator suggested he write an epitaph for Joe. The senator provided a pencil and a brown paper bag – of the type designed to carry a half-dozen bottles of Guinness – and after some thought, Gogarty wrote:

> Here is my tribute to 'lectrician Joe,
> Who fell to his death through the O in OXO,
> He's gone to a land which is far far better,
> And he went, as he came, through a hole in a letter.

Niall met Gogarty at the height of his fame as a talker: 'I was to see (and hear) him in action many times but it is difficult to convey his impact. His sharp tongue made many enemies, and some of his medical colleagues never forgave him. Asked for his opinion of Dr Ashe, a pompous Dublin physician, Gogarty snapped back: "I diagnose *folie de grandeur*. Ashe thinks he's the whole cigar."'

Niall, an astute literary critic, found Gogarty's novels 'flabby, verbose, and untidy', but when subjected to the discipline of rhyme and metre 'his genuine lyric gift found expression in a handful of near-perfect poems, and the flavour of his wit is preserved in a number of incomparably bawdy limericks'. Niall recounted a gathering at Gogarty's Ely Place home in the early 1930s:

> As the guests moved around in groups, two figures stood apart at the end of the room – George Russell (AE), deep in thought, murmuring into his great beard, and Yeats, head thrown back, his hand beating time in the air as he chanted some verse to himself. His arm rose and fell, the great ruby signet ring winking and flashing like a heliograph. What occult message was it signalling? What was afoot between the mystic and the poet? Were we witnessing the birth of yet another Byzantium poem? Could the Second Coming be upon us? (They were, in fact, discussing the last line of a Gogarty limerick.)[27]

On a sun-drenched day in Monkstown under cherry blossom, destined to bloom for no more than three weeks each year, I see Niall in splendid form, displaying his literary virtuosity to a group comprising Stephen Lock and Richard Smith (editor and deputy editor respectively of the *British Medical Journal*), myself, Monica and Tona. Niall rose with his glass and asked if any of us was aware that the inspiration for the closing lines of 'Ringsend' was Lapsang Souchong tea, once a most popular beverage in Dublin:

> And up the back garden
> The sound comes to me

Of the lapsing, unsoilable,
Whispering sea.

He went on to marvel at the power of the written word, so elusive but, when right, so beautiful; how to hold it once found, like mercury in the cup of one's hand, and how to thread the words into the needle that is art. By way of example, he compared the first published version of Yeats's 'Leda' in *To-morrow* in 1924 with the revised version published in *The Tower* in 1928. Were they, he asked, the same poem?

Although I failed to motivate Niall to write his memoir, I did motivate him to contribute an article for the *British Medical Journal*.[28] I was astounded by his phenomenal memory, enabling him to write the entire piece without recourse to quoted works. In this article, which is one of the finest written about medicine and literature, he singles two figures for primacy in the pantheon of doctor authors: Sir Thomas Browne (1605–82) and Anton Chekhov (1860–1904), to whom he pays the homage, 'Here, surely, untouched by dogma, is a secular saint, the most attractive personality in the whole history of literature.'

I often discussed Samuel Beckett with Niall, but strangely, he did not share my enthusiasm for his writing. He didn't believe Beckett's fame would last, except for *Waiting for Godot*. He regarded Brian O'Nolan as a greater writer 'whose sadness made Beckett look like an optimist'. He regarded *The Third Policeman* as a great work, 'revealing the schizophrenic aspects of O'Nolan's personality'. Niall believed that 'Brian had accepted that *At Swim-Two-Birds* was his greatest work and for the rest of his life was frustrated by knowing that he could never write anything better – his hate for the work was, therefore, understandable.' Niall thought he was unhappy sexually, being probably impotent. One evening we met his brother Michael O'Nolan in Goggin's and discussed the 'brother industry' and Michael's own work – the Irish 'La Guernica' on the Famine, which he would not allow anyone see. Niall explained that he refused to permit publication of his correspondence with Brian because, in the interest of economy, they wrote their replies on the same sheet of notepaper, and since many of the subjects in their correspondence were now respectable matrons of the establishment, publication might be embarrassing.'

We discussed the mixed reception of *The Plough and the Stars* in the US in October 1976. Niall thought it wouldn't have been a success without Siobhan McKenna and Cyril Cusack because they were constantly endeavouring to upstage each other. He recalled that in the French production years earlier, Cusack decided his stage departure would depend on his making an adroit stoop to snatch up his sash (dropped with purpose earlier) while uttering his closing lines with a flourishing exit. On the last night, McKenna upstaged him by standing on the sash, halting him midway through his exit. One critic had described this manoeuvre as the 'smartest piece of footwork since Gentleman Jim boxed Bob Fitzsimmons in 1897'.

Sylvia Beach stayed with the Sheridans for the opening of the Joyce Tower in 1962. When Niall discussed her upcoming interview, Sylvia showed him the notes she intended to read. He tore them up. Talking would not be her problem, he reassured her. How right he was. She spoke for the entire programme, with short interludes from Niall. She described her meeting with Joyce, the difficulty of publishing *Ulysses*, the occupation of Paris and its liberation, her imprisonment by the Germans, and post-war Paris with its French, American, English and Irish literati. She touched on her relationship with Adrienne Monnier, who helped found her famous Shakespeare and Company bookshop in 1919. During the 1920s, the shops owned by Beach and Monnier were across from each other on rue de l'Odéon in the Latin Quarter. Monica showed me a letter from Monnier describing the suffering she endured from being constantly aware of the sound of her blood rushing through her head. This was a form of Ménière's disease, and it ultimately led to her suicide. Malcolm Arnold, being party to this conversation, added that Bartók suffered a similar affliction – his hearing became so acute that 'he could hear insects when walking in the woods'. Beach died three years after the interview in Dublin, and although she had promised most of her Joycean possessions to Niall, they disappeared after her death.

I close this homily to Niall with sadness and misgiving, sadness at not having assisted him more in securing a visible place in Dublin's literary pantheon and misgiving for my failure to do justice to his gregarious and witty presence. I loved him dearly and owe him much. I hope that by recounting our many conversations, I will have assisted in our often-stated ambition to 'cheat the gods'.

Niall introduced me to a sector of literary society that included Mervyn Wall, Fanny Feehan, Roger McHugh and Michael Scott. But, most notably, he initiated my long friendship with Denis Johnston when he arranged for us both to attend a private viewing of the interview he had conducted on television with Johnston years earlier. After that, I became very friendly with Denis, and we met often to discuss his writing and his philosophy on life, which intrigued me. His quest for a deeper meaning to existence was apparent in some of his plays, but was expressed especially in the philosophical exegeses of *Nine Rivers from Jordan* and *The Brazen Horn*. His anguish on entering Buchenwald in *Nine Rivers from Jordan* allows the reader to share some of his pain in witnessing the atrocities the Nazis perpetrated there.

One evening at dinner we discussed Beckett and Joyce. Denis expressed irritation at the Joycean influence on Irish literature: 'In much the same spirit, whenever anything out of the ordinary appears hereabouts in print or on the stage, there is always some character who may be relied on to observe that it is influenced by our own local boy, Joyce.' I suggested that however one might wish to deprecate the Joycean influence, it was difficult not to liken Lucky's soliloquy in *Waiting for Godot* to the stream of thought in *Finnegans Wake*. Did Johnston go on to say Beckett would prove a greater intellectual force than Joyce? 'This nuisance is particularly rampant in the case of Beckett, who was, of course, Joyce's powder monkey for some years and attended the obsequies known as *Finnegans Wake*. Yet Joyce never had either the economy or the discipline to write a respectable play. Nor was he a thinker, as Beckett clearly is.'

In my discussions with Denis on theatre, we would certainly have talked about *Godot*, but I don't recall him making the analysis he expressed forcibly and presciently in an earlier comment:

> In short, Mr Beckett is no simple arithmetician and is not attempting to say anything so banal as the fact that two and two make four – or even five. His play is algebraic in that its characters have the quality of X. And what X means depends not upon him but upon us. If you feel that the point of this life – the intangible for which you may be waiting – is God, then indeed you may accept that solution as your X. If, on the other hand, you feel no such thing, then the play can still have validity in other terms.[29]

I looked after Denis and witnessed his declining health as the fate about which he had written with dread in *In Search of Swift* descended upon him. I was also in mind of his sceptical regard for physicians: 'Man would be frantic without the gift of death; as it is, he normally lives for something less than a century, and he does his best to make sure that this natural span is not enlarged into too long a senility, thanks to the efforts of his medical advisors.' Tona and I visited him and his wife, Betty, in a nursing home in Killiney, where they lived out their last days. On these occasions, I wished that medicine had advanced to permit the dispensation of a gentle potion to allow for a dignified departure.

On 8 January 1977 I drove Niall and Monica and John Ryan to Arland Ussher's residence in Blackrock, where he held an open house every Sunday. The only courtesy expected was that guests would bring a bottle of wine. I suggested bringing good wine, but John and Niall insisted Arland wouldn't know 'the difference between piss and wine' (and judging from the vintage on offer, they were probably right). We brought some bottles in Goggin's and arrived at the house where we were admitted to the living room. I recognized Seán Ó Criadan, Paddy and Nicola Bowe and Jeremy Williams (who had been keen members of the Victorian Society to which I once gave a lecture and, come to think of it, they about comprised the entire audience). Ussher's recently acquired wife, Peg Keith, was a vivacious woman in her early sixties who did all she could to put me at ease by pouring me a glass of sweet plonk for which, nonetheless, I was grateful.

Monica had told me ahead of the evening the background to Ussher's recent marriage. With his new wife, Peg, Ussher blossomed. It was rumoured that even his wig had benefited from his increased libido.

When the introductions were over, Monica addressed Peg: 'Of course, I knew Arland's first wife very well, and wasn't he so lucky to find you – how did he do it?' Peg took this with dignity, saying she also knew Arland's first wife very well. In fact, she'd been devoted to her, having nursed her during her illness and, in doing so, had fallen in love with Arland. Such was his first wife's regard for her, she would have approved of their subsequent marriage. 'Well,' said Monica, 'aren't you the little dote.'

I discussed books with Seán Ó Criadan, who was a serious collector. Niall, sitting on a 'milking seat', chatted with Ussher, who reclined in an armchair elevated on a dais so he had a view of the assembly and they looked upwards to engage with him. I observed Ussher without him being conscious of it. He was tall and fresh-looking for his seventy-seven years. Dressed in a herringbone tweed suit, which had the look of an unmade bed, he reminded me of a colonial gentleman who had seen better days. Yet there was none of the arrogance of that breed. His face was aquiline, not strong-featured yet interesting; he was bespectacled and smoking curiously – not inhaling – merely putting the menthol-tipped cigarette to his mouth, taking in a little smoke and exhaling immediately; this he must have done often since his fingers were nicotine-stained.

After a while, I was summoned to take the 'milking seat', and after a few hesitant moments, the conversation between us flowed surprisingly well, according to Niall and Ryan, who later commented that Ussher, being reclusive, was slow to make friends and warm to conversation. I asked him if he considered revising *The Face and Mind of Ireland*. He agreed that it merited revision but didn't think anyone would be interested in doing so. We discussed the short-lived magazine *To-morrow*, to which he had contributed, and the reasons for having to publish it in Manchester.

I mentioned the high regard I had for Beckett. He shared my admiration but only for the earlier prose. He thought *Godot* would have limited popularity for a short time. He didn't see Beckett as a lasting literary force but as one who would always have a small, devoted following. He added, 'Beckett's departure from Trinity did not cause a stir – there or anywhere else in Dublin – he was totally unknown at the time!' I suggested that some of Beckett's writing might have been influenced by *Finnegans Wake*, which led him to describe that work as 'Joyce's game'. I pointed out that, whereas Joyce had mastered the long and tortuous sentence, Beckett had conquered the short and stripped sentence. This amused him. 'One must turn to Proust,' he said, 'for the ultimate in mastery of the long sentence.' Why had Beckett not done more serious criticism? Ussher asked. 'His *Proust* was good, and he should have done more. His plays were quite awful, including *Godot*. Why should anything have to happen twice on a stage – this was going beyond the beyond.'

At this point, I asked, 'Do you like Beckett as a person? 'Oh yes,' said Ussher, 'very much. Marvellous character – could be great company but, on the other hand, could sit in company for hours on end with his head between his hands. If he was in that sort of mood, one left him alone; that was Sam!' 'I heard Beckett wasn't the life and soul of the party. Was he good company?' 'That depended on the party,' Ussher said. 'Beckett had always been a deep thinker, interested in the methodology of suicide. He often spoke at length about it, discussed performing it when his mother finally died, and he would be free to do so. But', he added with a mischievous glint in his eye, 'that was some time ago – I suppose he hasn't had time to get round to it.' He felt Beckett was full of gloom, and he did not think that there was humour in the later works. I suggested that the character of Belaqua had similarities to Jesus, which provoked the response, 'No! Jesus gave us hope – Beckett does not!'

I recognized a painting on the wall by Cecil Salkeld and mentioned my admiration for Salkeld's portrait of Con Leventhal which I had seen in Paris.

I knew from Con that Ussher was one of the few loyal friends who visited Salkeld during his illness. He said with sadness, 'I was very fond of Cecil, for whom I had great admiration.'

John Ryan and Jeremy Williams joined the conversation, and Ussher produced a manuscript of short pieces he had written mostly for *The Daily Telegraph* over the years. There were many essays, all typewritten, with the title 'The Limited Dog' taken from the first piece, an essay on the dog show held at the RDS on St Patrick's Day in the days when that feast was alcohol-free in Ireland except for the gathering of canine devotees. Ryan took the manuscript, promising to give it to his publisher. I suggested the title might be 'The Face and Mind of Arland', which Ryan later told me might have offended Ussher but that it was just the title needed. The evening ended around 12.30 am when we all bade farewell to our host and hostess with urgings to call any Sunday.

I never did revisit the Usshers. Betty Johnston related an amusing vignette one evening in Sorrento Terrace. She regarded Ussher as a good actor with a wonderful sense of humour, readily demonstrated when he played to a meagre matinee audience in a theatre in Dún Laoghaire. The play involved a bedroom scene, which required Ussher to sit in a dressing gown on the side of a bed where a woman lay. To alleviate the boredom on this particular afternoon, Ussher climbed in beside the astonished and furious actress who could do little about it. When Hazel Ellis, who had a lisp, appeared as the French maid with a letter on a silver tray, announcing, 'Monsieur, a letter for thou,' Ussher replied, 'Ah, *French* letters, I presume.'

The mention of Hazel Ellis reminded Niall of a ruse he and Brian O'Nolan had devised in an idle moment when they had started a fictitious correspondence in *The Irish Times*, choosing addresses and names from *Thom's Directory*; one of the names they had chosen was Hazel Ellis, and when the real Hazel Ellis wrote renouncing the contents of the letter, O'Nolan dared to write back claiming that he was the real Hazel Ellis and that the recent contribution was from an imposter. At this stage, the editor, R.M. Smyllie, spotted the ruse and, after discussion with the two miscreants, it was agreed that future contributions from O'Nolan would be submitted under the pseudonym Myles na gCopaleen.

I met Seán O'Faoláin in January 1977 after his lecture in the RDS, 'The Art of Writing'. I didn't get the opportunity to talk to him about his philosophy or challenge his pejorative views on the intelligence of artists. Concentrating on the short story, O'Faoláin acknowledged the imperative to write: 'Writers write because they must, they have no choice, but the obsession does not necessarily make one a good writer. The writer must make sacrifices. The writer has the exhilaration before starting to write, but he has to sublimate or extinguish the self to prevent himself from interfering with his fiction.'

O'Faoláin believed that the writer was intellectually privileged and 'differed from other artists, such as painters, by being an intellectual, which was why painters (like women) were such good company. They are not, generally speaking, intellectuals.'

Having succinctly and adroitly dispensed with painters – and women – he went on to define that 'the most important attribute for the short story writer' was 'the objective correlative' initially proposed by T.S. Eliot, in which in the reality of life was 'the event, which was often subconscious, that would stimulate the fiction'.

To illustrate this, O'Faoláin related a story from when he was lecturing in America. Students would bring short stories to him for comment; on one occasion, a Miss Anderson brought him a short story, which was awful. Not wishing to say too much about it, he asked instead about her home life. She came from a small town to which she would return when she had experienced 'life' at the university. Two weeks later she brought him another short story in which she likened the loss and nostalgia of leaving university to that of leaving home to come to university. She related this nostalgic coincidence to the point of departure and return on the railway track. The piece was so good that O'Faoláin thought it was plagiarized. When he mentioned his scepticism, she explained that the first story she wrote was before 'I cut my wrists.' O'Faoláin maintained it wasn't that the suicidal gesture stimulated her to write a better short story but that the suicidal gesture gave her the objective correlative, which then became the theme for leaving, and returning, home.

'The good writer never narrates; essay writers do that,' O'Faoláin stressed. 'Colette, a wonderful short story writer, said: "never narrate".' He referenced Henry James, a writer who hinted at but never described events, and Tolstoy (whom O'Faoláin regarded as somewhere 'between Beethoven and God, in terms of genius), who, with unerring authority, captivated his reader. But for O'Faoláin, one of the greatest short-story writers was Chekhov. He read 'Sasha' and then analysed the details Chekhov invoked without ever describing events.

Returning to the objective correlative, O'Faoláin read one of his popular stories, 'The Fur Coat', about a wife who always wanted a fur coat but, when she got the money to buy it, no longer wanted it. This story was written in 1932, but the objective correlative occurred in 1922 when O'Faoláin went for a drive in a friend's car with a RIC sergeant. They paused at a stretch of beach, and the scene made O'Faoláin remark, 'Wouldn't it make one love a swim?' to which the sergeant replied, 'Well, go ahead, have one.' However, O'Faoláin, noting it was cold, said, 'No, I don't have togs.' The sergeant helpfully added, 'I have a pair in the car.' O'Faoláin, having now decided against a swim, said, 'Ah, no. I don't think I'll bother,' which made the sergeant utter the objective correlative that was manifest those years later in 'The Fur Coat': 'The trouble with you bloody Irish is that you're always hankering after something, but when you can have it, you don't want it.'

Taken aback by O'Faoláin's view of painters as being intellectually inferior to writers, I met Niall Sheridan and John Ryan afterwards to discuss the lecture. Niall tended to agree with O'Faoláin (and noted that Salvador Dalí would have concurred),[30] but made an exception of John Butler Yeats, who once said: 'A work of art is the social act of a solitary man,' a sentence matched in his view only by Blake's declaration that 'the lust of the goat is the bounty of God.' John Ryan, himself a painter, couldn't agree with O'Faoláin. He remembered the young Seamus O'Sullivan telling him that when he was having his portrait painted by John Butler Yeats, who worked slowly, he stated that he was fearful of missing the last tram to Drumcondra, whereupon Yeats put down his palette and with an incredulous look asked, 'My God, do people actually live in Drumcondra?' And artists were not devoid of caustic wit. O'Sullivan, in his cups at the Stephen's Green Club, greeted his fellow artist Leo Whelan with: 'Ah, here comes the portrait painter who paints one posthumously.'

Apart from writing, John Ryan was an accomplished painter. He gave me an inscribed copy of *Remembering How We Stood* (or, as one wag dubbed it *Forgetting How We Staggered*) when it was published in 1975. We often discussed this account of the characters who had given Baggotonia its unique spirit and considered its adaptation for theatre. John showed me a draft with a scene in McDaid's depicting the conversational virtuosity of the imbibers who would later retire to the Catacombs, where 'the gathered pseudo-intellectuals in one corner would discuss Mahler's Ninth Symphony and the collapse of the Faustian culture, whereas the geniuses of Dublin – Kavanagh, Behan and O'Nolan – would exchange expletives and opinion in another'. Unfortunately, John's drama never found its way onto the stage.

John and I often discussed his plan to open an art gallery in Monkstown, which he eventually did. I bought paintings from him over the years, and we visited art exhibitions. Gene Lambert's first exhibition in the Project Arts Centre comes to mind. I purchased *Dolls* for £60, which was not the most pleasing painting visually but showed talent and potential for development. Niall Sheridan opened the exhibition, remarking that Gene had the best start in life that an artist could hope for: expulsion from the National College of Art and Design for being 'rude and insubordinate'. He went on: 'Such is the name of the Lambert family that one cannot be blamed for assuming that the world consists of "Lamberts" and "the others" and if one is fortunate enough to meet the Lambert family en masse, one forgets "the others".' He closed with characteristic humility: 'When I am dead and gone and forgotten, I know I shall have one small claim on history: I opened the first exhibition of one of Ireland's most famous artists.' The omens were deemed propitious when the President of Ireland, Cearbhall Ó Dálaigh, purchased *The Bicycle* for Áras an Uachtaráin.

Later we met Charles Brady, whose exhibition I had seen in the Caldwell Gallery and disliked. Brady, who was drunk, dismissed all Irish painters as 'being of little consequence to the world of art'. When I expressed admiration for Jack B. Yeats and even greater esteem for the father's portraiture, Brady declared that I knew 'fuck all about painting'. My obsession (along with the Irish intelligentsia) with literature had resulted in the suppression of, and neglect of, the painter. 'What of Jack Yeats?' I asked. 'Balls,' cried he, 'an impotent brush with little originality who rates only in the minds of philistines like you.'

He departed when Monica told him he was destined to destroy himself with booze. I visited Brady days later at his home in Dún Laoghaire to collect a painting I had purchased at an exhibition. The picture shows a simple pencil casting a subtle shadow. I regarded Brady as one of the promising painters in Ireland but found him disappointing as a person.

In 1976 John Ryan issued invitations to Con Leventhal and Sam Beckett to a meeting planned for a future Bloomsday in Dublin. I knew Beckett wouldn't attend. John remarked that Anthony Cronin thought Beckett would come to collect 'the divvies on the GSR (Great Southern Railway)'. He maintained that the Beckett family had leasehold interests in properties on the old Harcourt Street railway line that ran close to the family home, Cooldrinagh, in Foxrock. John dismissed the notion as typical of Cronin's cattiness, which led to a discussion on Cronin's commentary in *The Irish Times*, claiming that nothing good had come out of Ireland since the foundation of the Free State and that our only hope for survival lay in the North. I added fuel to the fire by mentioning a review in the *Honest Ulsterman* written by one 'Jude the Obscure' claiming that Cronin's *Dead as Doornails* and *The Life of Riley* were comparable to the writings of Proust, which infuriated John. The only explanation for such an outrageous assessment, he said, was that Cronin was none other than 'Jude the Obscure'. The discussion moved to a play of Cronin's staged years earlier at the Eblana Theatre. John thought it was a tedious ordeal, and afterwards he and his wife, Dee, met Cronin at a party where Cronin accused her of not paying attention to what he was saying, whereupon she reminded him, 'You had two and a half whole hours at the Eblana to say to me and the rest of the world whatever you wished and having listened to the crap you did manage to concoct, it is now most unreasonable of you to inflict yourself on me once again.'

In another conversation John recounted how he had narrowly escaped being knocked down by a cyclist on the East Pier. He recognized his assailant as the eighty-year-old poet Monk Gibbon. Niall chirped in that he regarded Gibbon as the greatest bore of all time. He had interviewed him for TV once and, just before the show, Gibbon said: 'Niall, what'll I do if I suddenly dry up?' Niall replied, 'Monk, if such an unlikely and happy event were to take place, we would see to it that at least a tablet, but preferably a marble monument, was erected on the spot to commemorate the auspicious occasion.' John recalled having reviewed some of Gibbons's books which he claimed were autobiographical and incredibly boring, with torrid love scenes enacted in 'the monkey's mind' but without sexuality, such as staring at a girl across the aisle on a bus. Niall recalled how Gibbon once interrupted Yeats when the poet was in full narration with a ringed finger held aloft, an event that made it necessary to usher a bewildered Gibbon away from the gathering.

In Goggin's one evening, John and Niall declared the subject of the evening to be Joyce's father, John Stanislaus, whom Niall had visited with Brian O'Nolan at 5 Claude Road, Drumcondra, in 1930 shortly before he died. The old man, who was in bed in hale and hearty humour, told Niall that 'Jim wrote quite well but was a poor storyteller and raconteur who had got it wrong in the graveyard in *Ulysses* where the two drunken men mistake the Virgin Mary for Mulcahy.' He wished James had devoted himself to developing his wonderful singing voice rather than writing books. When Niall visited Joyce in Paris, Joyce was appreciative of his visit to his father, who died a year later in 1931. He remarked that 'his father had been a raconteur par excellence who had influenced his powers of observation considerably'. I expressed my annoyance at the poor treatment Stanislaus Joyce received in the biographies of his son. John was enthusiastic about writing a book on Stanislaus Joyce and, after a few more pints, declared it 'the only book left that was worth writing'. Niall closed this by voicing a suitable epitaph for Joyce, who, after completing *Finnegans Wake*, declared: 'I can now do anything with words.'

Brian O'Doherty and I were brought together by our mutual admiration for Samuel Beckett. We first met over a decade ago when Brian, and his wife, Barbara Novak, joined me and Tona for dinner in Monkstown and our friendship grew in strength over the years. Brian O'Doherty lived most of his life in New York, where he established an international reputation as an artist and critic. However, his formative years can be traced to Baggotonia. He was tutored in medicine at UCD, then based in Earlsfort Terrace, and received practical clinical instruction in St Vincent's Hospital overlooking St Stephen's Green. He qualified as a doctor in 1952. Newman House, where James Joyce had studied some years earlier, was home to the Literary and Historical Society, where he listened to lively debate from many colourful personalities on diverse subjects that included a dissertation from Alexander Fleming on the forthcoming era of antimicrobial therapy. The artist Jack Yeats persuaded him to abandon medicine and devote his life to art.[31]

In 2016 *The Crossdresser's Secret* was published but received little attention as a result of inept publishing. It is a remarkable book which, in my opinion, surpasses his earlier novel *The Deposition of Father McGreevy*, that was shortlisted for the Booker Prize in 2000. In the same year, Brian reviewed my book *The Weight of Compassion and Other Essays*, which is revealing, not for what he says about me, but in that it identifies values and ideals in medicine that he espoused. For example, he deplored the loss of cultural appreciation in doctors:

> Have doctors lost their culture? ... I remember sophisticated cultural chatter over the operating table; occasional visiting physicians who knew more than a bit about music ... If your surgeon reads Proust, does that mean he'll operate on your gallbladder better than someone who doesn't? Not necessarily, but at least you have something besides your missing gallbladder to talk to him about when convalescing.

Brian identified early influences that encouraged his future life: 'Bethel Solomons, a remarkable Dublin Jew, whose sister, the painter Estella and her husband, Seamus O'Sullivan, bridged my divided loyalties (to the two trades, medicine and art) around 1950.' Brian goes on to provide an atmospheric flavour to these early influences:

> James Starkey edited the luxurious *Dublin Magazine* where he (far too kindly) published my (hopefully forgotten) juvenilia and invited me to tea ... His wife I met with pleasure, for I knew her paintings well – forceful, compositionally daring, overdue for revaluation. A sense of otherness, it seems, is inseparable from what is called 'the Jewish experience' – not unknown to outsiders and minorities of every kind. The otherness was probably emphasized during the reign of Archbishop John Charles McQuaid who proscribed the faithful from studying at the Queen's College, Trinity (including, by virtue of parental conformity) me.

In September 2015 I visited The Painted House (La Casa Dipinta), a house belonging to Barbara and Brian in the small town of Todi in Tuscany. Throughout the house Brian has created rope drawings and innovative paintings in vibrant colour paying homage to favourite themes, such as the ancient Ogham alphabet. La Casa Dipinta is a popular tourist attraction and visitors can apply for a guided tour.[32] The arrival instructions from Brian were clear:

> Get the Sulga bus for Pian di Porto, Todi, where Marco di Lernio will meet you. He will bring you to the Cesia hotel at the centre of town. Room 125 is reserved for you for two nights. The receptionist learned about Sam Beckett at school and is deeply impressed that you were his friend. Bon voyage – we are thrilled you are coming!

The citizens of Todi had affection for Brian and Barbara O'Doherty. When I joined them for coffee in the town square, a polite queue formed at the table so that the town's residents and some passing tourists could shake their hands. This process, which took hours, exuded reverence and affection. During my visit to Todi, I appreciated how much Brian and Barbara loved each other. I cherish many photographs of them, imagery that transcends prose in portraying this love.

Brian was an accomplished choreographer who could direct complex enactments from faraway New York. The most telling was the burial of his own alter ego, Patrick Ireland, in IMMA on 20 May 2008. At the interment site, a modest pine coffin holding a death-mask of the artist was lowered by pall-bearers into the ground. The sombre services included orations and poetry readings by prominent art world figures, culminating in a haunting recitation of keening, the traditional Irish mourning wail, by artist Alanna O'Kelly. 'We are burying the hate in a ceremony of reconciliation celebrating peace in Northern Ireland,' Brian stated. This 'joyous Wake and Burial', as the invitation and programme declared, was an unexpected coda to an event that took place thirty-six years earlier. On 30 January 1972 – a day now famously known as Bloody Sunday – a group of unarmed civil protesters, several of them teenagers, were shot down by British troops during a march in the Northern Irish city of Derry. Brian explained to me the creation of Patrick Ireland, the most famous of his many pseudonyms:[33]

> My mother's family were very much involved in the War of Independence and I suppose I am a Republican at heart but when the Derry massacre took place in 1972 and the paratroopers shot down those innocent people, I was in New York and I said, What can I do? I can't do anything, I can't throw bombs, I can't do things like that, but I said I cannot make art because if you make political art, you are always preaching to the converted, but I said I can change myself, I can give myself an identity change and I can become a living person whose very existence is a rebuke in the witness to what happened back then. So I took the name Patrick Ireland. Patrick because when the young man went for construction work in Britain, they'd say, 'Alright, Paddy. How are you, Paddy? Hey, Paddy.' It's not unaffectionate but it is ethnic. And the other thing I said is what do the British not want to hear? What's the last thing you want to hear about if you are English? It's your dark side, your bad conscience, it's that blot, out there on the left so I said I will call myself Patrick Ireland.

In 2011 Brian phoned me from New York and asked me to participate in a piece of theatre he was writing, *Hello, Sam.* I sent him a text message written as though I was having a short posthumous conversation with Beckett. I met Brian with Barbara in the National Gallery of Ireland, where I read this piece into a tape recorder. Some days later, hooded figures assembled in the Campanile of Trinity College. Accompanied by a large following, this procession marched through the campus to join a busy and bewildered multitude of rush-hour Dubliners at Lincoln Place before proceeding to the National Gallery. Brian's choreographed performance around a bog-embalmed figure suspended by ropes was enacted over several days according to a finite rhythm.[34] In a dimly lit corner at the periphery of the central room, the audience could listen to recordings by me, Anthony Cronin, Jota Castro and Michael Colgan, talking, as it were, to Beckett.

When Hume Street Hospital closed in 2006, its inner-city premises were sold, and part of the proceeds were used to establish the Charles Institute of Dermatology in UCD. A feature of this imposing building was a large, windowed foyer that begged for a statement. Accordingly, Brian was commissioned to install a rope drawing entitled *The Arrow of Curiosity, the Curve of Conciliation, and the Line of Inquiry*, in keeping with the scientific mission of the Institute. During the installation on 21 June 2011 I interviewed Brian about his past associations with his alma mater, UCD,[35] and how he had been influenced by John Butler Yeats, whom he had visited frequently in the Portobello Nursing Home, where the artist spent his last years, and about the many alter egos he had created. Brian's reminiscences of the artistic milieu that was Dublin of the time and the influences that led him to abandon medicine provide intimate details on this important period in his life.

In the competitive milieu of Manhattan, Brian challenged the conventions of modernism to become one of the most respected leaders of postmodernist art, or as one commentator put it: 'Few artists since Marcel Duchamp ... have pushed us so hard or given us so much to digest ...' The renowned artist George Segal hailed his work as 'the greatest oeuvre of drawings by any post-War American artist'. This statement exemplifies the fate that seems inevitably to befall our exiled artists – the land of their adoption claims them often for no other reason than the land of their birth forgets them. If ever there was truth in the aphorism of a prophet not being acceptable in his own land, Brian is an example *par excellence*. I proposed him for the Ulysses Medal, the highest academic honour that UCD can bestow on those whose work has made an outstanding global contribution. My application was declined, not once but twice. Perhaps even more surprising was my failure, along with other supporters, to have him awarded the Presidential Distinguished Service Award for the Irish Abroad, an honour reserved for Irish people living abroad who have achieved distinction to the credit of the country. None of this diminished Brian's affection for Ireland. He returned to his homeland often and always with generosity, as is exemplified in the magnificent gift of the Novak/O'Doherty collection of post-War American art to IMMA, named jointly with his wife, Barbara Novak.

Brian and Barbara O'Doherty were inseparable, with one giving to the other in art and life. Since their marriage in 1960 after he succeeded her as television lecturer at the Museum of Fine Arts in Boston, she has selflessly sublimated her career to propagate his, believing his art to be more valuable than hers. Barbara continues to paint beautiful flower studies and wrote not only the art criticism for which she is renowned, but drama and novels, one being *The Ape & the Whale*, in which her fascination with Melville is apparent. The O'Dohertys reserved a plot beside Melville's grave in the Woodlawn Cemetery in New York. When Barbara told me about this arrangement, by which she will be close to the shades of the two men she admired, I couldn't help suggesting that the achievement might lend itself to posthumous promiscuity, to which Brian quipped, 'but I will always be on top'.

Brian O'Doherty died in New York at the age of ninety-four on 7 November 2022.[36]

I met Petr Skrabanek when we worked in the Richmond Hospital in the 1960s, sharing an interest in neurology. Exiled from revolutionary Czechoslovakia, he fell in love with Ireland for the beauty of its landscape, the personality and generosity of its people and, above all, for its language, both native and acquired. He came to the Aran Islands with no money, no prospects and little English but soon mastered Irish and became intoxicated by the literature, including *Finnegans Wake*, on which he soon became an authority.[37] After qualifying in medicine, he joined the Department of Community Health in TCD in 1984 with a grant from the Wellcome Foundation. Here he flourished, bringing the warmth and breadth of European culture to Irish scientific research, a quality the Victorian clinicians had valued but one that had been squandered at the turn of the century. With the spirit of European iconoclasm, Skrabanek kept the medical evangelists in their hot boxes, choosing to take the broader intellectual view of a profession in disarray, a profession in need, moreover, of careful watching. Over the years, he became internationally renowned for his outspoken views on many popular policies, especially when they restricted people's freedom. The essence of his philosophy is in *Follies and Fallacies*, which he wrote with James McCormick, and *The Death of Humane Medicine and the Rise of Coercive Healthism*.[38] Though we diverged, he to epidemiology and the critical examination of medical dogma and I to cardiology, we never lost contact. We indulged from time to time in whiskey and tobacco but above all in conversation, and often exchanged comments on each other's medical and literary publications.

In 1992 Skrabanek invited me to be involved in translating *Les Chants de Maldoror* by Isidore Lucien Ducasse, otherwise known as the Comte de Lautréamont, published between 1868 and 1869. Aware that French and English were not his native languages, Skrabanek forged an intellectual alliance with Richard Walsh, a linguist and phoneticist, and the renowned composer Gerald Victory.[39] This eccentric trio pursued their mission in a window recess of the Leopardstown Inn, a suburban hostelry at the foothills of the Dublin mountains. They assembled there every Saturday at the stroke of 11 am, week after week, month after month, with their dictionaries, drafts of the translation and stacks of notes strewn on a table and enveloped in a cloud of tobacco smoke; they worked until 2 pm, on the stroke of which pints of Guinness and glasses of Crested Ten were ordered to facilitate a summary of the morning's work. Then, sadly in October 1992, to quote Skrabanek, 'Dick [Richard] decided to die.'

I came into the picture in 1992 when Skrabanek asked me if I would publish *Maldoror* under the Black Cat Press imprint. I was introduced to Gerry Victory for the first of many enjoyable sessions in the Leopardstown Inn. Apart from delighting in Ducasse's inventiveness and wonderful prose and agonizing over the nuances of a word, often for a whole session, we began to give more time to discussing the ultimate publication of *The Cantos*. By this time, I had entered Skrabanek's typewritten text into the modern contraption (as he called computers). He was anxious for the book to be illustrated, and I commissioned five paintings from John Long, a young artist whose work impressed me.[40]

Then cruel destiny intervened. One day in 1994 I was surprised to see Skrabanek walking along a corridor of Beaumont Hospital. A look of profound sadness filled his eyes as he told me he had just been diagnosed with advanced cancer of the prostate. We went down the corridor silently, an arm across each other's shoulder as I led him to have the investigations that confirmed the worst. We now met in Skrabanek's home rather than the Leopardstown Inn, where his wife, Vera, served coffee and chocolate biscuits. Gerry and I watched our friend sink rapidly, but he never relented on Lautréamont. My last memory is of his wasted body smothered by an enormous dictionary on his lap, the paroxysms of pain only quenched by the continuous infusion of analgesia, but he would transcend the misery of illness triumphant as the word that had eluded us sprang from the dictionary and his smile derided the apparent hopelessness of his condition. He died peacefully on 21 June 1994 at the age of fifty-four. Gerald Victory and I met on a few occasions to finalize some editing, and then Victory died on 14 March 1995. So Ireland lost one of its finest musicians, and I wondered if Maldoror was not striding across the plains of Erin and heading in my direction. But, not being given to superstition, I returned to *The Cantos*, checked the numerous corrections that adorned the many versions of the text and completed the editing with Vera. The Dublin *Maldoror*, as I have called this translation, joins four English translations of *Les Chants*.[41] However, I remain guilty for failing to fulfil my promise to Skrabanek to have his *limae labor et mora* published.

Sadly, my next association with Skrabanek was a posthumous defence of his reputation. His acerbic writings were challenged with vituperative detraction. He was accused of being in the pay of the tobacco industry, a 'paid stooge' to quote just one libellous condemnation from *The Guardian*, but, of course, the dead have no defence against libel. I examined the three 'tobacco-related pieces' to determine how Skrabanek earned his allegedly ill-gotten gains. In a letter entitled 'Smoking and Coronary Heart Disease in Women', he criticized a *Lancet* editorial for having accepted without adequate epidemiological evidence an association in women who smoked fewer than fifteen cigarettes per day. In the letter 'Penalising Smokers and Drinkers' (co-authored with James McCormick), Sir Raymond Hoffenberg is taken to task for suggesting to a House of Commons Select Committee that smokers and alcoholics should contribute towards the cost of their treatment because their abuse placed a large financial burden on the NHS. The Dublin correspondents, alarmed at the pernicious implication of such influential reasoning if it was to be applied more broadly, for example, to AIDS and intravenous drug abuse, reminded the president that tobacco tax alone raised a sum equal to one-third of total NHS expenditure annually. 'Smoking and statistical overkill' is a paper guaranteed to delight or irritate, depending on the reader's point of view, but, in either case, it cannot fail to excite admiration for its incisive erudition, laced with wit and humour.

In it, Skrabanek attacks the use of alarmist tactics by doctors, the media and politicians who manipulate statistics to scare the public, which, apart from being a ploy often based on falsehood, is clearly ineffective. By way of many examples, he cites WHO's dire admonition that half a billion of the world's population will be 'killed' by tobacco. All of which ignores another side to the equation that, as Skrabanek puts it, 'even if everyone smoked, that would hardly put a dent in the world population, which is increasing by a million every four days'. He appeals against the use of large denominators to make a case, such as the WHO's statement that over 100 million acts of sexual intercourse take place daily, resulting in 910,000 conceptions and 356,000 cases of sexually transmitted diseases – 'just in one day!'

There is a passionate plea in this paper for the downtrodden, the ill and infirm, the poor and uneducated, all lost in the bottomless sea of epidemiological statistics. Can the epidemiologists tell us, he asks, how to advise a 65-year-old widow with rheumatoid arthritis who smokes fifteen cigarettes a day? 'For many people, whether soldiers, prisoners, loners, bereaved, the elderly, or the unloved, a cigarette may be the last friend and solace.' He concludes with a plea for the human rights of the disadvantaged of society, those who are in danger of being isolated as 'pariahs' in the face of the seeming rectitude of 'responsible' citizens, who have the educational and general wherewithal to comply with the exhortations of the medical and political evangelists. *The Lancet*'s enquiry into the posthumous allegations vindicated Skrabanek, concluding that 'gadflies should never expect a friendly reception; Plato's associate Socrates suffered a more drastic form of peer review.' Seamus O'Mahony, a strong supporter of Skrabanek, acknowledges that, whereas there were occasions when his penchant for a cigarette may have influenced an occasional elision of evidence (such as his denunciation of passive smoking), he created a unique niche for himself as one of medicine's great doubters, 'an outsider on the inside'.[42] Skrabanek will be remembered when the many who rose up against him with unfounded invective are long forgotten. Ireland and the world of medicine is the better for his having had to find sanctuary in Ireland, a country he came to love.

Gerald Dawe came into my life as a patient with 'a touch of blood pressure' in 2001.[43] The patient/doctor relationship receded as our mutual love of literature became the dominant force in our friendship. We took a keen interest in each other's writing, and for me he brought the assurance of an academic who knew the world of literature intimately. We admired Beckett's unrelenting determination to explore the philosophy of existence and define the human condition. Sometimes, during a consultation, I had to remind myself that a therapeutic decision must override the literary discourse. This conflict of purpose led to our friendship being conducted on two interrelated planes in that the enjoyment of artistic endeavour was tempered by an appreciation of the transience of life. We shared the imperative to leave an affirmation that one had existed. There are contrasts that might have diminished Gerald's influence in my life. He is a Northern Protestant, and I am a Southern Catholic. He is an accomplished essayist, critic and poet. I cannot vie with Gerald here, but I can appreciate his poetry much the same way as I can relish music without being able to read a score. Indeed, his insight into the pantheon of poetry, especially the work of Sylvia Plath and Derek Mahon, has led me to look afresh at the poets whose voices have shaped his thoughts. Plath emerges as the dominant force in Gerald's poetical philosophy; his first published poem 'I'm Through' was heavily influenced by her style:

> It always happens like this,
> In a closed room, like a mouse
> Skittering about the floor.
> It always happens like this,
> so I was told.

There are different personas in Gerald, each the consequence of past circumstances, mainly where he found himself at different stages in Ireland. His writing could be a tale of three cities: Belfast, Galway and Dublin.

The Gerald I met first was a Trinity academic; competent, assured, often frustrated and not at ease with the academic demands of teaching and administration in a large university. As our friendship grew, I became aware of Gerald, the protestant Northerner whose great-grandfather was an Orangeman:

> The teacup shakes
> from stiff gloves
> he has on as
> the banner unfurls
> to a swaying scene
> of Slave and Queen

Gerald, the Northerner, is a restless soul, critical of the present and disturbed by a turbulent past: 'Relics of wars – statues, regimental flags, commemorative plaques outside churches, remaining blitzed sites – the whole business of destruction, sacrifice and loss were embedded in that civic world.'

Music was Gerald's escape from a troubled city. Van Morrison and The Beatles feature in his writing with adolescent passion. 'Music,' he wrote 'meant as much as writing. In fact, it probably meant more'. There is more to this than Gerald appreciates. The poet in him was drawn to the poetic harmony of song lyrics.

Gerald's schoolboy taste in reading was unusual:

> I read until I was almost blue in the face everything by Jean-Paul Sartre and Albert Camus and considered that my earlier experience had been what every good existentialist knows to be an encounter with the Absurd. If Roquentin, Meursault and Mathieu, leading figures in Sartre's fiction were not exactly role-models for a Belfast Protestant teenager with a paltry attendance at Sunday school and church, who was supposed to know any the different?

Belfast remains home, if not 'the' home for Gerald. Once out of Belfast, he was adrift: 'We did not belong anywhere else in Ireland; once out of Belfast we were effectively in no man's land.' He has spent most of his life in the no-man's land of Dublin and Galway, where he met his wife, Dorothea Melvin. Gerald, the Galwegian, is perhaps the most contented 'self' of these personas, at least for a time. Galway gave him freedom from the city of his birth, but at a cost. The geographical relocation 'produced an odd kind of divided self ... I often walked about almost in a trance'. Or,

> Who can tell, coming back and forth
> to discuss the place as if it were
> something
> different from that face in the unlit hall?
> The child will breathe easier and couple
> soon sleep the sleep of the Just.

He was confused by geographical contrasts: 'For much of the early eighties I was sleep walking, living and raising a family, and writing about the west of Ireland; learning about different styles of life and witnessing the saga of the North as it unfolded before a bewildered Republic.' But these transient influences of time and place make Gerald who he is: one with absolute subservience to the dominance of poetry, which he has protected from distraction. He pays tribute to this guiding philosophy: At certain periods of history it is only poetry that is capable of dealing with reality by condensing it into something graspable, something that otherwise couldn't be retained by the mind. He has acknowledged this aphorism (of Joseph Brodsky's) in ten collections of poetry.

Gerald the poet is undaunted by modernity. Morrison gave him the initial courage not to be fearful of modern-day expression, 'then Morrison's example kicked in very strongly, and the fact that he'd written about places, the streets and avenues of Belfast that I myself knew. It was almost as if a light went on and I found myself writing a whole sequence of poems about Belfast.'

Gerald is not afraid to embrace new words, concepts and forms of expression. Take, for example 'East Pier':

> Along with the sprightly
> There's one or two giving out,
> On the latest iPhone,
> Unassuageable complaint.

Or 'House of Fiction':

> The V-neck gansey,
> All in readiness for
> Princess Maud's heave
> Through the Irish Sea.

Sylvia Plath astounded Gerald when she demonstrated in one explicit stanza that poetry did not have to be restrained by niceties and convention; 'Death & Co' made him exclaim: 'You can actually say that in a poem, really?'

> The other does that
> His hair long and plausive
> Bastard
> Masturbating a glitter
> He wants to be loved.

The ordinariness of life permeates Gerald's poetry; take as an example 'Selfies':

> I look in the mirror
> And my mother looks back,
> The fall of the nose, brown eyes.
> For her too there's a grandmother lurking –

Gerald will be remembered not only as a poet but also as an essayist and critical commentator. *The Sound of the Shuttle* (inspired by Keats, who visited Belfast in 1818) and *The Wrong Country* chart not only the Troubles but cast a critical eye on poetry and literature. These sallies into the socio-political life of Ireland are testimony to Gerald's sensitive conscience reaching for a solution to the human condition in all its bewildering manifestations.

Our patient–doctor relationship soon led to literary collaboration. Our first venture was an essay I contributed to *Beautiful Strangers: Ireland and the World of the 1950s.*[44] This publication allowed me to pay tribute to shades from Baggotonia: Con Leventhal, Niall Sheridan, Denis Johnston, Micheál Mac Liammóir, Samuel Beckett and Nevill Johnson. Our next literary collaboration was a book of essays.[45] Gerald mercilessly and rightly stripped out the essays on medical institutes, which I had been trying to force into a book in which they had no place, and edited the entire collection, giving *The Weight of Compassion & Other Essays* an order it lacked. He was drawn to the book since much of it was in keeping with his own literary philosophy; he wrote in the foreword:

> The torment that afflicted so many during the twentieth century – from the persecution of the Jewish minority of Europe to the abominable legacy of landmines in our own day, to the current plight of medical doctors in Bahrain, to the bureaucratic and social struggle for a 'fit-for-purpose' medical system in

Ireland is viewed with hope, commitment and, critically, an energetic enthusiasm that inspires with its social democratic vision of what makes a decent egalitarian society possible.

Our next endeavour preoccupied us for over two years. After Con Leventhal's death in Paris in 1979, I visited his partner, Marion Leigh, in boulevard Montparnasse. On one of these visits she gave me a case of papers, diaries and notebooks with the admonition, 'you will know what to do with these'. I filed them away with similar archival material except for one notebook with poems written by Con's deceased wife, Ethna MacCarthy. MacCarthy had been a friend and confidante of many intellectuals in TCD, including Beckett, Con, whom she would eventually marry, and Denis Johnston. I found the poems remarkably passionate but, needing enforcement for my view, I turned to Gerald, and he rekindled my enthusiasm. *Ethna MacCarthy: Poems* was published in 2019. Gerald puts MacCarthy's poetry into contemporary perspective:

> It was in the mid-to-late 1940s that MacCarthy hits her stride as a poet with several very moving and self-confident poems. The decade sees the writing of 'Lullaby', a truly remarkable poem which foreshadows the exposed lunar and death-haunted landscapes of Sylvia Plath's poetry by well over a decade later.[46]

Gerald remains in my mind's eye as a poet of optimism who has made the tedium of existence more pleasurable by believing that the human spirit can overcome the vicissitudes of a world in turmoil:

> Dear God, but isn't it great to be
> sitting by an opened window,
> on the day of your birthday,
> birds singing to their heart's content.

Robert Ballagh has been my friend for ever. Our childhood paths crossed in Baggotonia, but our interests in painting, Beckett, and our mutual friendship with Brian O'Doherty, brought Tona and me into regular contact with him and his wife, Betty. Ballagh is a talented artist and a delightful companion who is never afraid to express his views on life and politics, often to the chagrin of conservative members of society. Ballagh was often in the company of David Davison, whose photography he admired. We spent time on joint projects, one of which was

The Beckett Country, for which Ballagh designed the maps that introduce each chapter; with Tona, he designed the special edition that Beckett signed. When UCD wanted to commission my portrait to acknowledge my contribution to developing dermatology in Ireland, I suggested Ballagh. The portrait now hangs – or should I say stands – in the boardroom of the Charles Institute of Dermatology in UCD.

Ballagh's colourful personality has attracted numerous biographical studies and he has written an outspoken memoir.[47] He remains a vocal critic of Irish society north and south.

The artist Harry Kernoff was ever-present in my Dublin of the 1960s. He was a frequent visitor to Roberts Café on Grafton Street. Kernoff always looked, as another put it, as if he had 'stepped from his bed into his hat'. Many years later, after his death, I visited his sister in her flat on Mespil Road with Colin Simon to advise her where she should place Kernoff's many paintings that were stored under her bed.

I met John Betjeman when he visited Ireland in 1976. He was no stranger to Dublin and knew Niall Sheridan and Denis Johnston, who had warm memories of him from the 1940s when he was known as Seán Betjeman. He was particularly friendly with Patrick Kavanagh, who paid homage to this former Dubliner with the immemorial lines:

> Show me the stretcher-bed I slept on
> In a room on Drumcondra Road.
> Let John Betjeman call for me in a car.
>
> It is summer and the eerie beat
> Of madness in Europe trembles the
> Wings of the butterflies along the canal.
>
> O I had a future.[48]

This would not be Kavanagh's only poetic reference to his friend:

> I have taken roots of love
> And will find it pain to move.
> Betjeman, you've missed much of

The secrets of London while
Old churches you beguile.
I'll show you a holier aisle –

The length of Gibson Square
Caught in November's stare.
That would set you to prayer.[49]

Tona and I were invited to meet Betjeman for afternoon tea at 'Clontra' in Shankill, then owned by the well-known medical Tomkins family.[50] The house, built on the shore, was designed by the eminent nineteenth-century architects Sir Thomas Newenham Deane and Benjamin Woodward in the Italian medieval style, and this was Betjeman's interest on that afternoon. When I told Betjeman I worked in the Rotunda Hospital, he deserted the guests and, sitting down with me, recounted his love for the hospital.[51] The Rotunda was one of Betjeman's favourite buildings, particularly the chapel. However, I was surprised when Betjeman said that, though he loved the architectural beauty of the building and the stucco splendour of the chapel, his most precious memory of the hospital was of the little wire cots that hung at the end of each bed, within easy reach of the mother's foot, who could rock her infant to sleep. Here, simple ingenuity and practical need were in harmonious accord. Every time I did my ward round, these cots reminded me of the memorable afternoon with Betjeman in Shankill.

That is, until one day I became aware that the wire cots had been replaced by expensive cots on wheels. This act of modernism, which not only made it difficult for me to listen to the hearts of mothers with my stethoscope, dispelled the feature that Betjeman admired. The usual calmness of my ward round was disrupted and the nursing sister guiding me to the patients in need of my attention, who also resented the change that had been made without discussion, told me with sadness that the wire cots had been thrown out. I went to the yard where refuse was dumped, and amazingly one wire cot lay against the wall having fallen from a refuse lorry. I retrieved it and it is now in the RCSI museum as a small memento acknowledging the sensitivity of the gentle soul that was John Betjeman.

Ben Kiely, a latter-day Baggotonian, became a dear friend. We met often, usually with Seamus Heaney, Christy Cahill (who lived with Ben for a time) and Kevin Cahill. There were many dinners in the RCSI where Kiely entertained in song and verse. He and his partner, Frances, joined my family for Christmas day in

1993 in our home in Clifton Terrace, Seapoint.[52] Ben had a prodigious memory, which with his repartee and willingness to break into song after a quantum of wine, made him delightful company. I collected him from his Donnybrook home one morning when he demonstrated how he set his burglar alarm – a garden rake laid prong-side up on the three steps leading down to the back door so that any would-be intruder would be knocked dizzy, if not unconscious, as they took their first nefarious step into the Kiely domain.

7. *Parisian Interlude*

who may tell the tale
of the old man?
weigh absence in a scale?
mete want with a span?
the sum assess
of the world's woes?
nothingness
in words enclose?
Samuel Beckett. 'Tailpiece', *Watt* (1953)

I visited Paris frequently between 1977, when I first met Samuel Beckett, and 1989, the year of his death. During this period he introduced me to his friends, some of whom, such as A.J. (Con) Leventhal and Edith Fournier, shaped much of my thought and writing. I have written essays and books on Beckett and Leventhal, and I have joined with Fournier in collaborative ventures.[1]

Con came into my life in the 1970s. He lived on boulevard Montparnasse with his partner, Marion Leigh, and whenever I visited Paris – often with Tona – we joined them for drinks in their book-lined flat under the watchful eye of

Cecil Salkeld's frame-flowing portrait of Con, before crossing the boulevard to La Coupole for dinner.

Con succeeded Samuel Beckett at TCD as lecturer in English and French in 1932. After the death of his first wife, he married Ethna MacCarthy, who had been a close friend of Beckett. Sadly, the marriage lasted only a few years because Ethna died in 1959 from throat cancer at the age of fifty-six.[2] Con retired to Paris in 1963 to assist Beckett by acting as a critical and erudite literary arbiter; he also threw a protective mantle around his friend, besieged, as he was, by so many admirers.

Apart from his erudition and knowledge of international literature, Con's most enduring characteristic was his humour. He was an exuberant conversationalist and was always delightful company. The characteristics that make the fictional Bloom of *Ulysses* so attractive were also evident in the persona of Con, who loved Dublin for its eccentricities, hypocrisy, humour and carefree nonchalance. Like Bloom, women were an essential ingredient of life, or as Niall Montgomery put it so pithily: 'Con had the great joy, all his life, of being cherished by beautiful and talented women.'[3]

In 1965 Con met Marion Leigh. She had been married to Walter Leigh, a prolific composer who was killed in action near Tobruk in 1942, just before his thirty-seventh birthday. Marion and her three children went to Canada to escape the London Blitz. She became a documentary film executive with the National Film Board of Canada and frequently visited Paris in this capacity. She told me that Con fell in love with her at a railway station, a version at variance with the account of her meeting him through Mavis Gallant, the Canadian writer and a mutual friend of Beckett's.[4]

I was at ease with Con's Judaism. Indeed, I had studied the influence of Judaism in life and art, which is a recurring theme in many of Con's articles and in his poetry. His appreciation of lesser-known writers such as Amy Levy and Hannah Berman was a characteristic of his literary awareness. Perhaps the intensity of his Dublin Judaism justifies Niall Montgomery's assertion that 'the Jewish community, at least in 1920s, exhibited the same sort of syndrome that was characteristic of the two larger groups: 'loyalty, orthodoxy, piety and the fiercest intolerance'.

I was introduced to Dublin Judaism at an early age. My first contact with a Dublin Jew was when I accompanied my father to Ballybrack to visit his friend Bethel Solomons. My memory is of a strikingly handsome man taking me by the hand down the long garden to his summerhouse where he was writing his autobiography, *One Doctor in His Time*. Solomons was a renowned Dublin figure who became the first Jewish Master of the Rotunda from 1926 to 1933 and served as president of the Royal College of Physicians of Ireland from 1946 to 1948. He earned ten international rugby caps for his country between 1908 and 1910. My father told me Solomons enjoyed recounting how one Saturday, after doing his rounds in the Rotunda, he threw his rugby kit into the back of a horse-drawn cab for the trip to Lansdowne Road where Ireland was to play England; en route he asked the driver what he thought of Ireland's chances, to which the latter replied: 'Ireland, Ireland – fourteen Protestants and one effing Jew and you call that Ireland!'

I succeeded Mervyn (Muff) Abrahamson as acting professor of Materia Medica and Therapeutics at the RCSI, when he departed Ireland to work in Israel in 1973. I then inherited his Jewish practice and came into contact with a diverse gathering of Dublin Jews and learned to admire their individuality even if, as an outsider, I couldn't fathom or integrate with their religion and customs. When I worked in Smethwick, I befriended another Jewish couple late of Dublin, Ivor and Phyllis Radnor, who became close friends to me and Tona. With this absorption in Dublin Jewry, it was hardly surprising that when I was invited to give the Leonard Abrahamson Memorial Lecture in 1986, I chose Irish Judaism as the subject for my presentation.[5]

Con and I shared another common bond – we were both unsuccessful publishers. I was attracted to his failed periodicals, *The Klaxon* and *To-morrow*. Con was the first to recognize how remarkable Joyce's *Ulysses* was – 'the riches are embarrassing' – but when he submitted a review to the *Dublin Magazine,* word came that the printers in Dollards would down tools rather than participate in the publication of the blasphemous writings of Joyce. In anger, Con wrote: 'A censoring God came out of the machine to allay the hell-fire fears of the compositor's sodality.'

Determined that his review would appear in print, he produced the delightfully outspoken magazine *The Klaxon*, which introduced itself in strident tones:

> We are the offspring of a gin and vermouth in a local public-house. We swore that we were young and could assert our youth with all its follies. We railed against the psychopedantic parlours of our elders and their maidenly consorts, hoping the while with an excess of Picabia and banter, a whiff of Dadaist Europe to kick Ireland into artistic wakefulness.

The Klaxon, lasting for only one issue, was not permitted to achieve its nobly stated ambition, but it did at least publish a truncated version of Con's article on *Ulysses*:

> In truth, there is no real parallel to Mr Joyce in literature. He has that touch of individuality that puts genius on a peak. Rabelaisian, he hasn't the joie de vivre of the French priest; Sternesque, he is devoid of the personal touch of the Irish clergyman. Trained by the Jesuits, he can't guffaw like Balzac when he tells a good story. He is a scientist in his detachedness, but *Ulysses* is, nevertheless, a human book filled with pity as with sexual instinct, and the latter in no greater proportion in the book than other fundamental human attributes.

After the demise of *The Klaxon*, Con launched another polemical magazine, *To-morrow*, which was to fare only slightly better than its predecessor in that it lasted for two issues, each of which had to be printed overseas to escape the moral rectitude of the Irish typesetters. Nonetheless, it provided Yeats, Francis Stuart, Lennox Robinson and Con, among others, with a platform from which they voiced with an iconoclastic honesty their stifled sentiments on art: 'We proclaim that we can forgive the sinner, but abhor the atheist, and that we count among atheists, bad writers and Bishops of all denominations.' Con delighted in these ostensibly failed literary eccentricities which, paradoxically, by being denied longevity, were able to attract the attention not only of a select readership in Ireland to what would have been seen as heretical dogma but were also assured a place in literary history.[6] Indeed, the intention of daring so assuredly to fail was a concept of achievement Beckett would duly espouse. Niall Montgomery put it nicely when he commented that 'these gestures were failures by the world's standards, but what a disgrace to our society if they had not taken place.' Con and I discussed compounding our mutual weakness as publishers by resurrecting the *Dublin Magazine*. We went so far as to agreeing to be joint editors, Con being based in Paris and me in Dublin, but he wisely decided against this initiative, reminding me of his past excursions into failed periodicals, adding that he also had some fiascos in business, having sold two libraries to establish an unsuccessful bookshop in Nassau Street. He opted instead to keep watch on my often-contentious role as editor of the *Irish Medical Journal* from which I was eventually fired. Unfortunately, Con was no longer with us to witness this debacle, which he would, no doubt, have savoured.

Con was probably happiest in the theatre. On stage, literary expression could be enhanced by innovative ingenuity. For fifteen years he contributed a quarterly

'Dramatic Commentary' to the *Dublin Magazine*. The first of the series appeared in the October–December issue in 1943 and continued until 1958. The strident tones, the felicitous style and discerning criticism that were to characterize this unique diary of Dublin theatre are evident in the opening lines of the first contribution:

> At its inception the Abbey Theatre incurred abuse to be followed by universal approval with a consequent acceptance at home like the prophet approved by proverb who only receives posthumous canonisation in his native town. Recognised in the first instance by the discerning few for the right reasons, praised by the equally discerning few in foreign parts, the latter brought their compatriots round to appreciation of a dramatic mode, which despite a regional language and local dramatis personae, succeeded in crawling out of its provincial rompers to an adult metropolitan influence.

He enjoyed acting and appeared in some of Denis Johnston's plays. His appreciation of theatre, his affection for Irish drama and his empathy with actors give his criticism warmth and feeling devoid of parochial sentiment. These qualities, together with his familiarity with European theatre and literature, make the *Dramatic Commentaries* a valuable legacy of theatrical criticism.

I shared with Con an intense admiration for Beckett's writing. What often struck me was that, deep though Con's admiration was for Joyce, Beckett's genius surpassed him: 'Beckett is in a sense a more intellectual writer than Joyce and his jousting with words has a background of erudition deeper; one suspects, than that of the master – the *cher maître* of the *avant garde* of the twenties and thirties in Montparnasse.' In Con's view, Beckett's abandonment of what had gone before, including the Joycean experiments with language, elevated him above the mightiness of his Parisian friend. Even if 'Mr Beckett's work is not for the many,' an appreciation of Joyce demanded certain preconditions: 'To appreciate Joyce fully one had not only to be a Catholic but to have a Dublin background in addition …' Beckett's refusal to conform, his desire and ability to lift literature from the abyss of convention, his audacity and courage in daring to go further than Joyce, were qualities that appealed to Con: 'It may well be,' he wrote of *Fin de Partie* in 1957, 'that there is still a public that believes the age of experimentation is not over, that profundity, however painful, is still preferable to vapid reiterations of tried and tiring formulae.' Above all, it was Beckett's ability to establish indelible points of departure in literature that most fascinated Con. '*En attendant Godot* belongs to no school, it will make one,' he wrote in 1954.

On his last visit to Dublin in 1979, it was clear that Con was dying from cancer. I accompanied him and Marion to Montparnasse to give him what solace I could. He died shortly afterwards. Much as I missed him, it was nothing to the loss Beckett felt. He lost his close friend and learned confidant, who protected him from the frivolous multitude clamouring at his door.

From having been a dominant intellectual figure in Dublin, Con was almost forgotten at the time of his death, even in TCD where 'he had once been a power in the land'. I was determined that this man of letters, who had been the first to praise *Ulysses*, who had written a criticism of Dublin theatre and who had been a formidable influence on one of the century's greatest writers, should not pass unnoticed into the mists of time. Two years after his death, I brought together a band of loyal friends 'to consider how best to commemorate his erudition, charm and literary influence'. We resolved to establish a scholarship to enable an Irish graduate student in English or Modern Languages of TCD to study in Europe. The Scholarship Committee was composed of myself and a band of Con's friends.[7] Beckett, whom I met regularly in Paris to discuss the scholarship, was an advisor and contributor to the auction. Con's friends and literary associates, and academic institutes at home and abroad contributed generously to the fund and auction, which was held in the Samuel Beckett Rooms in TCD on 15 March 1984.

When the executive members of the scholarship committee met in my home to decide on how best to apply the funds, it was seen as fitting to celebrate the occasion with liberal potions of Jameson whiskey. As the evening wore on, John Jay, a solicitor who had been a racing buddy of Con's, proposed that, in keeping with Con's love of racing, we should put the entire proceedings from the scholarship venture on a 10/1 outsider at the forthcoming Galway races, and either establish a really worthwhile scholarship or be excused for having made a damn good effort to do so. Paddy McEntee finally persuaded us against this option, happily for over thirty recipients of the Leventhal Scholarship who have travelled to various parts of the world to further their studies.[8]

Con's reputation was international. He was in demand as a critic and much of his erudite commentary is to be found in *Hermathena* (the TCD magazine), the *Dublin Magazine*, *The Irish Times* and international newspapers such as the *International Herald Tribune* and *The Financial Times*. He was also a regular broadcaster for Radio Éireann and the BBC. Niall Montgomery gives us a tantalizing prospect of hidden gems: 'We don't know what creative work of Leventhal's remains unpublished, but we do know that he published in *Hermathena* some fine translations from the French … He translated Valéry, Eluard, Supervielle …' The essays, translations and criticism buried in archives merit publication so that his writings can be reassessed and enjoyed. I hope the archive I have established in his name in the Library of TCD will serve as a potent point of commencement for such scholarship.[9]

Edith Fournier was a close friend for over thirty years. We first met in December 1989 at the Sainte-Anne Hospital to which Samuel Beckett had been transferred following deterioration in his health in Le Tiers Temps, a home for elderly people, where Edith had cared for him and where I had often visited him.[10] Edith had also looked after Beckett's wife, Suzanne, who died on 17 July 1989.

Beckett requested that Edith receive one of the special editions of *The Beckett Country*, which he signed on its publication to honour his eightieth birthday in 1986. Likewise, I was aware of Edith's long association with Beckett, and we were delighted to meet at last.

Following Beckett's death, Edith and I became close friends, and I visited her often in Paris, firstly when she lived in a tiny one-roomed flat on rue Amyot. Some years later Caroline Murphy, who was Beckett's niece, appreciating Edith's past kindness to Sam and Suzanne and the importance of her role as a translator of his work, arranged for her to occupy a more spacious flat on 26 rue des Cordelières, where she spent the rest of her life. She cast her critical editorial eye over the books and essays I was writing on medical and literary subjects. She translated the essay 'The Weight of Compassion' into French[11] and joined with me in co-editing Samuel Beckett's unpublished first novel *Dream of Fair to Middling Women*,[12] which had been written at the Hôtel Trianon, on the rue de Vaugirard in Paris during the summer of 1932, when the author was twenty-six. Beckett asked me to publish the novel, which he referred to as 'the chest into which I threw my wild thoughts' but not to do so until he was gone 'for some little time'.

When Jérôme Linden granted me permission to edit *Dream* for publication, I realized it would be a more complex task than I had originally envisaged. I asked Edith to join me in the undertaking, knowing that her linguistic skill and appreciation of the young writer's boundless literary repertoire would protect the exuberance of youthful genius that permeates the novel. The first edition of *Dream* was published by the Black Cat Press in 1992 with a foreword by me and Edith, and a revised edition was republished by Faber & Faber in 2020.

When I first met Edith she had an academic appointment at the Sorbonne University, but she resigned shortly thereafter. She augmented her small pension by reviewing texts submitted for publication to Irène Lindon at Les Éditions de Minuit and, although she translated other authors,[13] her main preoccupation was translating Beckett's works into French.[14] In later years she developed an innovative technique for producing attractive computer-generated images to illustrate the covers of books for Les Éditions de Minuit.

Edith often shared with me the difficulties she had interpreting Beckett's elusive text for translation. She was a superb linguist, but translating the poetry and phraseology in Beckett's writing was often complex. In writing *The Beckett Country*, I had come to appreciate that Beckett sometimes modified the meaning of English words with an 'Irishness' that made finding translational equivalents difficult. She had moments of translational despair when the French equivalent of an English word became almost untranslatable.

Some random examples from her correspondence relating to the translation of the poems illustrate her meticulous search for the meaning of a particular word, but also her reluctant doubts about the merit of some of Beckett's poetry. 'Serna III' and 'Enueg I', for example, presented several difficulties:

> Dear Eoin, … If I understood what was said about the Merrion Strand on that web site, it is where a very small river flows out into the sea. Do you know the name of that small river? It is not the Tolka, or is it? Could you please send me, if it is no trouble, your beautiful photograph of 'the fingers of the ladders hooked over the parapet, soliciting' of 'Enueg I'. Back in 'Serena III' is there any way of finding a view of Misery Hill (with or without its phallic 'arch-gasometer')? If it was called a Hill not only by Sam, why so? Whereabouts was it situated in the docks?

Likewise, the poem 'Dortmunder' from *Echo's Bones* didn't lend itself to ready translation: 'Many thanks for your email. I quite agree with what you say about "sustaining the jade splinters". Do "Madams" pick up their "customers" in the street? I am deeply grateful for your so patient and precious help. I still have one or two lines to try and improve, and then I'll send the whole thing to Irène [Lindon].' Beckett himself was aware of the challenge she faced in translating *Echo's Bones* when, with a laugh, he wished her 'fun and luck' to manage the translation. Edith persisted and concluded: 'I shall never know if I have "managed". I have only done the least worst I could.'

Translating 'Whoroscope' (or WHORRENDOUSCOPE as Edith called it) was a frustrating undertaking. She wrote:

> What do you think of 'Whoroscope'? Do you like it? I see it as a young student's over pedantic prank. Am I completely wrong? Can you understand why it won the prize for a poem on the subject of time? I realize we are in 1930 at a time when the ambient breeze is wafting more or less pungent whiffs of Surrealism and Dadaism all over the place, in literature as in art. … 'The shuttle of a ripening egg combs the warp of his days' could, as the whole poem, be illustrated with Dada or Surrealist art (I do like very much some of it, do you?), for instance, amongst others, with Max Ernst's (whom Sam liked) paintings and drawings, or a few of Picabia's early paintings. In some ways, *Whoroscope* is Descartes being shredded through a dadaist/surrealist mincer. Or am I straying?'

I replied, admitting my reservations about the poem:

> Yes, to be frank I never understood *Whoroscope*, but I don't hold myself alone on that. Perhaps the judges felt the same sense of bewilderment but knew they were dealing with talent! He certainly stepped into the surrealist movement with relish but did not linger, don't you think? A bit like his dabbling with Joyce and then getting as far away from his style, as distinct from his genius, as possible. In fact, *Whoroscope* smacks much of *Finnegans Wake* in style. I suppose he had to dabble in Dadaism, just to get it out of the way.

Edith responded:

> Yes indeed, Sam dabbled in Surrealism but then distanced himself from it completely, as almost all of the Surrealist painters did too. He also distanced himself from Joyce, taking exactly the opposite direction. Fortunately, he found out that he did not need to follow in anybody's footsteps, and he hated any 'school' of thought. I believe however (but I may be wrong) that, later on in life and in his works, he did create a thoroughly new 'surrealism' of his very own, far away from all the trappings, dogmatic paraphernalia and distasteful rites of the erstwhile literary Surrealism with a capital S. Unfortunately, the word *surrealism* has been kidnapped and lastingly branded by André Breton & Co. Lacking therefore the free, untainted use of that word and for want of a better one, I would venture to say that, in his later works, Sam has created a brand-new *hyper reality* the likes of which there is no echo to be found in any other literary work, and a few but very few echoes to be found in works of art.

Biographical details on Edith Fournier simply do not exist. She was an intensely private person who believed that her life was of no relevance and that after her death, her presence would be of even less consequence: 'To sum it up briefly: in so many ways my life has been only an almost life. Hence, perhaps, my ingrained nobody-ness ...'

But there are contradictions to this appeal. Firstly, she assisted me with this memoir by editing early drafts and the final text owes much to her critical advice. I asked her to allow me include a brief account of her life, if for no other reason than to prevent erroneous speculation that would do a disservice to her, and to her fascinating family. She wrote: 'I know full well that if my background needs ever to be mentioned somewhere, then you are the one and only person who can do so correctly, in the most tactful, most discreet way.'

Despite her reservation about leaving any trace of her own or her family's past, Edith made a film on her parents. She asked for my advice on this project in which she had used early film from her father who had acquired one of the first movie cameras. The final nostalgic tribute showed the influence of a coterie of brilliant colleagues and friends who had been dominant figures in her family background. Edith gave the film a haunting poignancy by her choice of background music: 'Where Have All the Flowers Gone' sung by Marlene Dietrich.

Yet another contradiction to Edith's desire for anonymity was her fourteen-page essay about her father, entitled 'Daddy-long-legs'. When I expressed my enjoyment of this sensitive production, she wrote: 'Of course, you are its first reader (and will be its only one I should think) and it goes without saying that I do expect from you, all along, the most severe comments and criticism, please.' I encouraged her to persist with her literary and cinematic *recherche du temps perdu* and she responded positively: 'I fear you are slightly too indulgent about my father and far too indulgent about my capacity to tell his story. Nevertheless, I have started trying and here is the rough draft of two first "chapters". I have not yet even reached his youth. I don't see how this can interest anyone but myself.'

When the intellectual brilliance of Edith's family led me to comment on the richness of her genetic legacy, I received an interesting riposte on genetic inheritance:

> Yes, my father was a remarkable person in so many ways and my mother was also a most remarkable person, perhaps even more so intellectually. But, is being remarkable a fact which one inherits straight away in one's genes? I don't think so. It is not bequeathed as an intact ready-made wrapped up whole gift. And it comes with the heavy burden of having to try and live up to it.

In disclosing these snippets, I realize that I am giving Edith a 'presence' rather than the 'nobody-ness' she yearned for and, that in doing so, I may offend her shade, which I will hasten to placate (along with my conscience), by recalling the pleasure it gave us both in her flat in Paris to mull over the pictorial and written material she rescued from various family troves and to reconstruct her past from the fragments (shards might be a better word) she had saved from obliteration.

Edith's paternal grandmother, Juliette Bonnet-Maury, was born in 1870 in Dordrecht, the eldest daughter of Georges Bonnet-Maury, a French Protestant clergyman who preached for a time in the Netherlands. He believed that the three monotheistic religious groups – Muslims, Jews and Christians – should be brought together, and he wrote numerous books in which he endeavoured to make his fellow Christians understand the Muslim and Jewish faiths. He was also eager to defend women's rights, maintaining that a woman should not lose her maiden name in marriage and be able to transmit it to her offspring. He decided, therefore, upon his marriage to Isabelle Maury, to change his own family name to Bonnet-Maury.

Georges and Isabelle Bonnet-Maury had two daughters, Juliette and Evaldine, and one son, Alfred, all of whom became staunch agnostics or atheists who adhered to a strict moral code. Edith's paternal grandfather, George (also known as Louis) Fournier, was born in Bordeaux in 1867, the son of a baker whose wife, Marie, was an illiterate pastry cook. He won state scholarships enabling him to study medicine at the Paris University. He worked in the Hôpital Cochin where he became head of the venereal disease department and he established a laboratory to develop new drugs for the treatment of infectious diseases, notably syphilis. This expertise allowed him to charge his wealthy patients lavish fees, thereby enabling him to treat the poor without charge.

In 1897 he met Marie Curie, with whom he formed a close friendship. She discussed her work with him, and he was a frequent visitor to her home. During the First World War he helped Curie organize a small fleet of radiography ambulances, one of which she drove to the wounded soldiers on the battlefields in 1914.[15] Dr Fournier's expertise was sought in Hungary, Austria, and the courts of Serbia and Russia. He befriended Tolstoy, who frequently invited him in the 1890s to stay at his home, Yasnaya Polyana, where he met scientists, writers and poets. Edith never met her grandfather, who died from cancer of the bladder in 1930, before she was born, but she did know his adoring wife Juliette Bonnet-Maury whose only child, Georges, Edith's father, was born on 14 September 1901.

According to Edith's notes, her father was pampered 'to a ridiculous extent'. He was intellectually precocious with a voracious curiosity. A subject, once understood, was soon dropped for another so that in later life he became 'a rather highly curious and inventive jack of all trades than a painstaking master of one'.

From early childhood Georges regularly accompanied his father to the Hôpital Cochin and a strong bond developed between them. He was allowed to skip several forms and entered university to study science before his sixteenth birthday. After graduation, he joined Marie Curie's scientific team at the Radium Institute where he met Edith's mother, J.S. Lattes, an innovative physicist, who was one of Marie Curie's assistant scientists from 1921 until 1936. She fell in love with and married Georges Fournier, and their child, Edith, was born on 24 March 1935.

The scientists in the Institute handled radioactive substances without being aware of the dangers of radioactivity. However, an entry in the *Science Newsletter* of 1926 is notable in acknowledging the contribution of Edith's parents to the dangers of radiation and the need for protection. 'Radium Gift Useful' reads:

> The gift of one twenty-eighth of an ounce of radium, worth $100,000, made by the women of America to Madame Curie in 1921 has been instrumental in establishing and proving a new law of nature. Mme. J.S. Lattes, a worker in Mme. Curie's laboratory has described in *Annales de Physique*, her studies of filtering radium rays. Madame Lattes was originally interested in finding the best method of wrapping up the applicator tubes which are brought in contact with the flesh of a patient who receives radium treatment, but her results led her into fundamental studies of the absorption of radium rays by different materials. She was able to confirm definitely, using the American radium, a law discovered by Georges Fournier in the same laboratory, according to which there is a simple mathematical relation between the absorption coefficient of a material and its atomic number. She also learned how to avoid the destruction of the flesh, or necrosis, which occurs when a radium tube is improperly used.

Remarkable though these observations were, neither of Edith's parents appreciated that the toxic effects of radiation would damage the foetus of a pregnant mother. Edith loved when her parents came to kiss her goodnight and waved their fluorescent hands, but she didn't know the price her body would have to pay.

The Curie and Fournier families worked closely on the rapidly developing science of radiation treatment in Marie Curie's Radium Institute, but outside the laboratory, strong familial relationships brought them close together. Edith wrote: 'I seem to remember that Eve [Curie] gives a lively description of the holidays they spent in Brittany … Eve mentions the people I often saw in my childhood: Jean Perrin, Charles Seignobos and André Debierne, and also, of course, the Joliot-Curies (Irène and Frédéric and their children Helène and Pierre) and the Langevins.'

Edith has commented humorously on her parents' somewhat unconventional approach to academic ritual:

> Here … is a 1922 photo of my mother sporting the appropriate garb for her Doctorate in Sciences, though with no water-bottle hat cum tassels in her eyes. I wouldn't put it past her to have lost the mortar-board in a café, though certainly not in such a wild place as a bar. No such photo of my father two years later on the same occasion. He was always very much of a rebellious creature. To don a doctorial gown was beyond his very scant ability to brook any conventional trappings. He attended the ceremony in his everyday suit, was accepted all the same, yet not without a good deal of reprobating eyebrow-raising and gruff-huffing from all the surrounding acaca assembly. The same sort of thing happened when, after the war, he was awarded the Légion d'Honneur. No sooner had the sparkling golden medal hanging on a large bright red ribbon been very ceremoniously pinned on his lapel than he availed himself of the very first opportunity to unpin it surreptitiously and thrust it into his pocket, thus sporting a barren lapel amidst the gathering of tinselly bedecked ones during the Elysee champagne dipping that followed. 'I'm not a Christmas tree,' he is reported to have remarked, a comment for which he later apologised.

It is evident from a childhood photograph of Edith that her knee bones were badly deformed and the skeletal deformities inflicted on her *in utero* worsened with age. Despite many orthopaedic procedures, her mobility decreased with advancing years and eventually she was confined to a wheelchair. As well as being unable to walk, she was in constant pain, which she tolerated stoically. During the last two decades of her life she was confined to her flat except for odd excursions to the little garden opposite the flat on rue de Cordelières in a mobile buggy, which I often manoeuvred from the basement of her building. Her sister, Stella, also brought her on outings when she visited her in Paris. On these excursions, she delighted in the fragrance of the flowers and the pleasure of breathing the spring air. Edith contended with these infirmities and never allowed pain to interfere with her work. Added to the skeletal deformities, she also developed hypertension and elevated blood cholesterol, which caused narrowing of the carotid arteries. I advised her on the most appropriate medication and donned my medical persona when I visited her. Although she drank little alcohol, she was a heavy smoker, but I overcame my medical instincts by not denying her this small pleasure.

In the last decade of her life Edith and Stella established a close friendship. Their father, Georges, joined General de Gaulle in London on 19 June 1940. Having tried unsuccessfully to get his wife and daughters to England, he deemed them lost and started a new family. After the war, it was agreed the two families shouldn't meet. It was only in 2011 that Stella's daughter Fanny managed to bring the two sisters together with the help of Les Éditions de Minuit accepting to forward a letter. Stella, who lived in the south of France, visited her frequently and supported her as her health declined. Stella's visits were a source of great comfort to Edith, and she became not only her confidante but also her means of egress from the solitude of her flat to the world of sunshine and flowers. Edith Fournier died on 24 April 2022 at the age of eighty-seven.[16]

Every time I write about Beckett, a simple but telling adage always springs to mind: 'One cannot explain the existence of genius. It is better to enjoy it.'[17] I was introduced to Beckett's writing in the 1950s when my brother Hugh recommended I read *Murphy*. At this time Beckett was relatively unknown but I became fascinated by his work and appreciated an innovative philosophy made tolerable by a characteristic of Irish humour that accepts the inevitability of tragedy in existence. But my medical studies kept me away from literature and I put Beckett aside for some years. Even in the 1960s when I was a student and later a house physician to Professor Alan Thompson, who had been to school with Beckett at Portora, the passport photograph of Beckett hanging in his office in the Richmond Hospital did not excite my curiosity. A decade later when I was a consultant physician, I had the sad duty of caring for Alan Thompson in his final illness in 1974. His death and Quaker burial prompted the first of many letters I would write to Beckett:

> His funeral devoid of all hypocrisy and cant, features so characteristic of our nation's obsequies – was a touching and strangely peaceful affair … The funeral at Temple Hill Cemetery had an ambience peculiar to Dublin – crisp air, moist mist insulating sound, muted feet on gravel and grass, and a spirit laid to rest with the dignity of simplicity – you would have approved. Few words for a man who used words sparingly but with great effect.

Two years later I wrote again to Beckett on the death of Alan's brother Geoffrey: 'I had a sad but beautiful letter from Ursula, who I have never met. What a pity Alan and Geoffrey were not allowed a little time in peaceful retirement.'

When my medical training as a cardiologist had been completed in Britain, I returned to Beckett's writing and to the secondary literature that his work was attracting from academic scholars, most of whom were not Irish. It seemed some fundamental characteristics in the Beckett *oeuvre* were being overlooked, namely an Irishness that was manifest in humour and dialogue, personality and place. I began researching – appropriately enough, on a bicycle – the topography of place and terrain and the inferences of subtle and often occult humour. I realized that much of Beckett's surrealistic prose emanated from the reality of Beckett's early memories of Dublin, which he had rendered unrecognizable in his creation of the 'unreality of the real'. When I discussed my reasoning with Con Leventhal, he arranged for me to meet Beckett.

My first of many meetings with Sam at the Café de Paris in the PLM Hôtel on boulevard Saint-Jacques was in October 1977. Our relationship, which began simply as one between a renowned writer and a devotee, would grow into a lasting and trusting friendship that can be traced in the evolving intimacy of his cards and letters to me over thirteen years.[18] This correspondence, compared to the lengthy and informative letters of his earlier years, was relatively terse – being often simply confirmation of the details of our meetings – but I was faced nonetheless with deciding on the future of these communications. I could have destroyed his letters, and he would have approved. He told me that the sluice in his flat was a convenient receptacle for the letters people had written to him and wished the same fate for those he had written to others. Nevertheless, I couldn't bring myself to destroy his letters and other personal papers.

Another option was to sell the correspondence, but that would be a betrayal of friendship and trust. I could have contributed my letters to *The Letters of Samuel Beckett 1966 to 1989*,[19] but I did not do so because the first editors, Martha Dow Fehsenfeld and Lois More Overbeck, ignored Sam's stipulation that only content referring to his work be published. He often expressed to me his regret at having given consent for the correspondence – 'I thought it would go around in circles for years – concentric spirals that would fizzle out.' On one occasion he phoned me from Paris to ask if he could divert the two editors of the correspondence to Dublin because he could not face meeting them as arranged in Paris. I agreed and organized access for them to the correspondence in the library of Trinity College and entertained them in Dublin as I would do on several occasions.

This was not the first time Sam would regret granting entrée to his private existence. He deplored having given the 'neither help nor hinder' acquiescence to Deirdre Bair for her biography. It has been argued (and I must admit, at times persuasively) that adherence to Beckett's stipulation to permit only references to his work would have denied access to the deliberations that beset a maturing genius at chronologically pertinent moments within the continuum of a long and productive life. These apparently paradoxical sentiments may justify a more open-minded interpretation of his directions for the annihilation of personal material. The final option open to me was to donate my correspondence to an academic institute and this is the course I have taken with all my Beckett material.

To return to this first meeting with Sam in the Café de Paris, I began hesitatingly by discussing Alan Thompson and my friendship with his widow Sylvia. Sam was interested in Thompson's achievements in the Richmond and his association with my father who, with Thompson, was one of three senior physicians on the hospital staff. This discussion went on at length and I wondered when I would be able to turn to his writing, which I had been told (erroneously as I would later learn) should not be an item of discussion unless broached at his behest.

Then suddenly he said: 'Con tells me that you are a cycling authority on the topography of my past!' I was able then to tell him how I had been visiting his old haunts in the Dublin mountains and on the coast of Dublin Bay. He warmed to the subject as I described what had changed and what remained the same. He closed his eyes as I journeyed from one location to another, pausing only if my description caused him to seek embellishment or if I needed to clarify a detail in his writing. He was not always able to do so because 'it was so, so long ago'. I went on to express the view that I thought various authoritative writers were doing his work a disservice by failing to recognize the relevance of place and particularly by their mistaken attribution of the reality of existence to imaginative unreality. When I described a Japanese treatise on the surrealistic interpretation of a passage from *Company*, we had the first of many chuckles in the Café de Paris: 'Nowhere in particular on the way from A to Z … As if bound for Stepaside. When suddenly you cut through the hedge and vanish hobbling east across the gallops.' We agreed that for the reader unaware that a place with the remarkable name Stepaside existed and given the context of the piece, a surrealistic interpretation was plausible. Sam intimated that the name provided a means for him to cast a mantle of unreality over the prose and we discussed how being Irish could be advantageous to the interpretation of some of his writing.

This first meeting concluded with Sam's approval of what I was doing, and he encouraged me to persist with 'the project', offering to help if assistance was needed: 'When coming to Paris, just make me a sign!' We parted on this happy note and my research now became more detailed, more purposeful. Sam's enthusiasm brought me to meet him more frequently at the same café. I recall those days of warm memories walking through the Luxembourg Gardens with 'Beckett on my back' – a heavy cache of photographic imagery for him to peruse. As my research progressed, he no longer needed to close his eyes to imagine the locations I had visited; we could examine the photographs I was unearthing from his childhood and the newer, sensitive landscape images that David Davison was creating. The photographs were often moments of enlightenment for Sam, and he would give me his memories of a particular place or person, Miss Elsner's school being an example. And the bicycles of childhood, or bicycles in general, were never far from conversation. He remembered his childhood bike in *Company* and the beggar woman: 'It happened, Eoin, I used to cycle to the Elsner school.' He frequently asked for details of my cycling trips around the Dublin mountains, and he often became quite engrossed in a particular place. He would send me away to explore details of place names around Foxrock. I recall him having a particular fascination for the name Ballyogan, which I researched in detail for him. I was careful not to trouble him for explanations of the obvious and there were times I had to leave the obscure anchored in obscurity.

Sam took mischievous delight in sending me cycling in search of odd locations, one such being Foley's Folly, which is central to the novel *Company*. I searched the local historical sources to determine its whereabouts without success until I located a place bearing the name Taylor's Folly in an Ordnance Survey map of the Dublin mountains. This ruin on the slopes of Two Rock Mountain, which had once been a farmhouse, now housed a drove of delightful pigs. The view, the overgrown nettles, the solitude (if you ignore the pigs) and the air of tranquillity all seemed to suggest Foley's Folly, but it was well out in the country, whereas Sam had written that the den was 'not in the country'. When I showed him David Davison's wonderful photographs of Taylor's Folly (and the pigs) he took time to marvel at the beauty of the place and the view of Dún Laoghaire harbour in the distance before saying: 'Eoin, it is beautiful, but I have never been there.' He admitted finally that Foley's Folly was Barrington's Tower, which was in a field very close to Cooldrinagh, but because there was 'no music in those words' he changed the name to Foley's Folly. Indeed, had I read his words carefully, I would have realized how much off course I was. But I did not complain. To cycle along those dear back roads that he had trudged with his father in all weathers, and when summer came, or even better, spring, it became 'a matter of some difficulty to keep God out of one's meditations'.

The Café de Paris could also be a place of poignant sadness. On one occasion after I had laid out the latest photographs that my research had unearthed, the image of Bill Shannon, the whistling postman in *Watt*, brought Sam to tears. I bid farewell by placing a hand on his shoulder to show I understood and left him to his reminiscences. This and similar moments in Paris have drawn me to the view once expressed by John Banville that 'Beckett is an old-style landscape painter.' Indeed, in a presentation with Margaret Drabble at the Enniskillen International Beckett Festival in 2013,[20] I likened Beckett to the Romantic poets, notably Wordsworth, portrayed with feeling in her book *A Writer's Britain*, and although the comparison was a revelation (to her and the audience), it can be supported in many passages of pastoral tranquillity in Beckett's novels and poems; for example, 'The Roses are Blooming in Picardy' in *Watt*, the spring evocation at the foot of the Dublin mountains in *More Pricks than Kicks* when it is 'a matter of some difficulty to keep God out of one's meditations', or the 'birdless sky' with 'the odd raptor' on the Dublin mountains in *Mercier and Camier*. Sam edified the landscape of his youth, and in his prose he immortalized the beauty of the Dublin mountains, just as Wordsworth did for the Lake District in poetry. James Knowlson alludes to a similar thought in his foreword to *The Beckett Country*: 'I have heard some Beckett scholars speak of a marked vein of lyricism in his writing about nature, while others have disputed whether one can speak of lyricism in the case of a writer who so drastically and so self-consciously deflates his own descriptive effects.'[21]

I have previously commented on how different Joyce and Beckett were regarding the memory of place as the stimulus for creative expression. Whereas Joyce is fastidious in securing detail from friends or *Thom's Directory*, Beckett doesn't generally pay attention to the accuracy. There is the hilarious exception when Sam asked Con to go to the GPO in O'Connell Street and measure the height from the ground to the arse of Cuchulain to determine if it would be possible for Neary to dash out his brains against the hero's buttocks. This aside, Sam is not concerned with embellishing reality. He is more concerned with letting the creation stand, unsupported in its own beauty; in his hands, it does so, whereas the expectation would be for it to disintegrate.

The most revealing instance is the revelatory moment on the pier with 'the foam flying up in the light of the lighthouse and the wind-gauge spinning like a propeller' when he saw 'the whole thing, the vision at last'. This is unmistakably the east pier of Dún Laoghaire harbour beneath the spinning anemometer (the exact spot has been commemorated with a plaque). However, when I showed Sam the photographs of the storm-lashed pier, he confided, in the tone of one who had pulled a fast one and is proud of it, that the revelatory moment when he 'saw the whole thing … at last' took place on the more humble pier at Greystones harbour on a black stormy night when he had walked to the sea from the house his mother had rented there.

What started as a humble notion of mine gained momentum with Sam's increasing interest, and the idea of a book began to evolve. Once we agreed that this was the objective, our meetings focused mainly, but not exclusively, on selecting the most appropriate images to illustrate his childhood and youth in Ireland, predominantly in Dublin. Our deliberations reached fulfilment in 1986 with the publication of *The Beckett Country: Samuel Beckett's Ireland.*

Although Sam alerted me to misinterpretations I might have made in the book, surprisingly he did not alert me to an important error I discovered years after its publication. The Grand Canal was familiar terrain for Beckett when he visited Jack Yeats in the Portobello Nursing Home and they would then walk along the canal towards Chapelizod when the older artist imparted an ethos that would greatly influence the young writer: 'He is with the greats of our time, Kandinsky and Klee, Bellmer and Bram van Velde, Rouault and Braque, because he brings light, as only the great dare bring light, to the issueless predicament of existence.'[22] This canal would provide the setting for what I believe to be the most beautiful lines ever written by Beckett. Sitting by a weir, Sam shared his mother's last hours as she lay dying in the Merrion Nursing Home overlooking the canal. Sam captures not only the sharing of suffering with his mother, but also the profound sense of loss, and relief that her suffering is over. He accepts the inevitability of death, the timelessness of age, the inexorable cycle of death and birth and life – in short, the melancholy state of existence:

– bench by the weir from where I could see her window. There I sat, in the biting wind, wishing she were gone. (Pause) Hardly a soul, just a few regulars, nursemaids, infants, old men, dogs …

– the blind went down, one of those dirty brown roller affairs, throwing a ball for a little white dog as chance would have it. I happened to look up and there it was. All over and done with, at last. I sat on for a few moments with the ball in my hand and the dog yelping and pawing at me. (Pause.) Moments. Her moments, my moments. (Pause.) The dog's moments.[23]

In *The Beckett Country*, I attributed this 'bench by the weir' to the Huband Bridge lock. Many years after the book's publication, I realized that the window in which 'the blind went down' could only have been seen from the weir at Baggot Street, not from the Huband Bridge. Why did Sam not alert me to the error? This may be an example of the irrelevance of accurate detail in that he cared little about which 'weir' inspired him; the resulting words were all that mattered; or it may have been that, as with Bill Shannon (the postman singing 'The Roses are Blooming in Picardy'), the moment evoked by the memory was too intense to countenance discussion.

Sam was aware that the book would be the most daunting publication undertaken by the fledgling Black Cat Press. I struggled with its structure but decided on the format during a fortnight of seclusion in the Tyrone Guthrie Centre at Annaghmakerrig.[24] I decided that a chronological imposition would not be possible, if for no reason other than Sam writing in his seventies was as likely to evoke memories from his first as from his eighth decade.

Structure was one thing, content another. I would rely on photography to illustrate the narrative, and Nevill Johnson agreed to my using his sensitive images of Dublin from the 1950s. David Davison accompanied me to the places around Dublin that inspired Sam's later writing. The portrayal of that land could be achieved only by an artist willing to familiarize himself with the terrain, its people and its fickle sky and light.

Bobby Ballagh agreed to create maps to illustrate the topographical nuances for each chapter and, with Tona, designed the limited de luxe edition. Gerry Dukes and Jim Knowlson read and corrected the proofs and Knowlson wrote the foreword, in which he made prescient observations on the influence the book would have on Beckett scholarship. Ted and Ursula O'Brien of the OBEN imprint devoted themselves to the design and typesetting of the book. I turned to the board of the Black Cat Press to obtain approval for the book as a project. Frank Pike at Faber & Faber agreed to a joint publication, albeit with Black Cat doing all the work and providing the financial backing. Since the text depended on quotations, permissions would have made the project prohibitively expensive, but Sam instructed his publishers to waive fees. I was aware that duotone reproduction of black-and-white photography was necessary for the beauty of the imagery to be transmitted to the printed page. At that time, duotone was not readily available in Ireland, so I engaged the Italian publisher Arnoldo Mondadori in Verona to print the book. I travelled to Verona and slept on a couch in the printing house so the printers could raise any issues they discovered as printing progressed. One issue was that if I persisted in blackness as dark as a pint of Guinness the ink would carry over to the opposite page. Another was an intentional question mark in a quote from *Watt* that was seen, understandably, as an uncorrected error.

I kept Sam informed of progress and he encouraged me to keep going. Realizing I was encountering financial barriers, he offered to sign a special edition to assist in overcoming these difficulties.[25] *The Beckett Country: Samuel Beckett's Ireland* was published just ahead of Beckett's eightieth birthday on 13 April 1986 and met with his approval: 'My gratitude to Eoin O'Brien, David Davison and their collaborators for this kindly light on other days.'[26]

During our meetings we discussed many topics, but I made few notes, believing that to do so was a betrayal of trust. We spoke often by telephone. As I look back on what notes I had taken, I am struck by a feature that seems strange in retrospect but at the time was accepted by us both as an integral part of communication between us. We often sat in silence, not talking for minutes but nonetheless communicating. When the silence was broken, usually by Sam, we carried on oblivious of the pause. Before parting, I'd help Sam put the whiskey, black pudding (from Tona) and some Irish newspapers (*Press* and *Times*) into the brown nylon hold-all he always had with him and which, when filled, drew the comment, 'All set with ballast like stonypockets'.

Sam became involved in the Leventhal Scholarship. He suggested it should not be restricted to Paris but that it should be extended to Europe and that it should be in modern languages rather than French and English. We discussed how much the scholarship might realize, and he made suggestions for membership of the committee and possible subscribers, particularly in the Jewish community. He promised to donate items and money for the auction; he wanted me to take a cheque for £500. I published a booklet in 1984 for the scholarship – *A.J. Leventhal 1896–1979: Dublin Scholar, Wit and Man of Letters* – and sent a copy to Sam. Some years later John Minihan gave me a photograph of Sam intently poring over page eighteen of this publication on which there is a double sketch of him by his friend Avigdor Arikha, the Romanian-born artist. We often discussed Con and he worried that Marion was missing him and that going through his papers and being in the flat on her own must be painful for her. We also discussed the service that was to be held for Con in TCD.

When I began *The Beckett Country* in 1975, I realized how deficient a book purporting to illustrate the origins of much of Sam's writing would be if *Dream of Fair to Middling Women*, a novel that ranks as one of his most Irish writings, was not carefully studied, and he agreed.[27] He agreed to my quoting whatever I thought relevant. My reading of the transcribed manuscript of *Dream* in the Beckett

Collection at the University of Reading was, of necessity, cursory at the time, but it led to many discussions about the work. In particular, Sam was interested in the reaction of a man more than thirty years his junior. His interest was more acute, I think, because he had forgotten much of the detail of *Dream* and our discussions allowed us to wallow in the nostalgia of his Dublin. We discussed his having 'pilfered' the 'chest' and whether anything worthwhile remained. I assured him the novel stood firm because, unlike the vignettes in *More Pricks than Kicks*, it had a beginning and an end, though we joked about the 'middle'.

At a meeting in 1986 he told me that he was giving serious consideration to publishing *Dream* so that he could help John Calder by giving him a text for publication, and he asked me for my thoughts. We bandied about the pros and cons. My recommendation was that he should publish it but when we next met shortly afterwards, he had made up his mind. He could not face the pain of going back to the 'chest' where the wild thoughts of his youth were securely stored. However, he told me *Dream* should be published, but not until he was gone 'for some little time' and he asked me to hold the 'key' to the 'chest' until I thought fit. Jérôme Linden, Beckett's literary executor and long-time friend, gave me permission to edit *Dream* for publication. Edith Fournier, who had translated many of his writings from English to French, joined me in the editing. Linden advised against launching the book when he realized that John Calder was going to dispute publication but, unfortunately, this request came too late. The fracas that followed led to a farcical publication fiasco in which Calder copied the Black Cat edition for an American edition in which he even included the foreword I had written without my permission. This sorry sequel in bringing *Dream* to the public was demeaning, but happily Faber & Faber have republished a pristine version of the book, adhering meticulously to the original Black Cat edition. I hope this novel will now find a new and appreciative readership.

Sam was fascinated by the concept of a photographic exhibition of *The Beckett Country*, which Jim Knowlson's wife, Elizabeth, had first suggested. *The Beckett Country: An Exhibition for Samuel Beckett's Eightieth Birthday* took place at the University of Reading in May 1986 and a booklet was published to accompany it. I sent this to Sam in advance of meeting him a week later in Paris. We sat in our usual spot in the Café de Paris and, after some pleasantries, he withdrew the book from a grubby brown bag. As he opened it, I realized that the popularly held view of his not reading what had been written about him would not apply to my catalogue. He opened it at page fourteen, saying hesitatingly: 'Eoin, I cannot reconcile a quotation from *Watt* with the original publication and I have even checked back to the manuscript.' Together we unravelled a curious happening. The piece of prose in *Watt* that describes Watt's journey on the train from Harcourt Street to Foxrock was read thus to me by Sam:

> The racecourse now appearing, with its beautiful white railing, in the fleeing lights, warned Watt that he was drawing near, and that when the train stopped next, then he must leave it. He could not see the stands, the grand, the members', the people's, so ? when empty with their white and red, for they were too far off.

The question mark, Sam explained, was a device he rarely used, perhaps only when he was so tired that he left it to the reader to devise the appropriate word. Unfortunately, an inventive typesetter in Reading remedied this deficiency by inserting the ridiculous and utterly meaningless words 'six chairs' for the eroteme; by doing so, the passage was rendered senseless but was alas in irrevocable print. I decided immediately to change my scheduled route from Paris to Dublin to Reading (much against Sam's wishes) where I tried to find the compositing genius without success, but I established with the printers that the proofs had been correct and that the published run of 1000 copies should be pulped and reprinted.

Initially Sam had not appreciated the size of the exhibition and he became intrigued by its design and layout. For the Paris exhibition, he wanted Jean-Louis Barrault and Madeleine Renaud to host the exhibition in the Théâtre du Rond-Point and had had a telegram from Barrault confirming his acceptance. He was worried the space would be inadequate to house the whole exhibition (this concern proved to be well founded). We compromised by omitting some of the panels. The exhibition was formally opened by the Irish Ambassador, Tadhg O'Sullivan. Sam was delighted that the exhibition had been shown in Paris and he sent a warm telegram: 'Dr. Eoin O'Brien, c/o Theatre Renaud Barrault, Ancien Theatre du Rond Point. De tout coeur avec vous tous. Sam.' Aer Lingus hosted a dinner after the exhibition in Fouquet's Restaurant on the Champs-Élysées. After the Paris showing, Sam continued to watch over the exhibition with 'fatherly affection'. He was concerned about it going to Madrid and Bonn without me accompanying it but was glad I could go to New York. He wanted to send telegrams to the venues to which the exhibition would travel. However, he could not face the intricacies of doing so and he asked me to convey his warm wishes wherever the exhibition went.

At a meeting in July 1977 after he had returned from Stuttgart, Sam was full of praise for German television, which, compared to the BBC, allowed him time 'to do the thing properly'. In defence of the BBC, I suggested that the BBC *Ghost Trio* was good, and he added that the Stuttgart production was 'about equal'. This meeting concluded with a discussion on 'But the clouds…' I commented on how marvellous a line it was, and he said it was one of Yeats's most beautiful poems, and he went on to recite the poem's closing lines.

Childhood often came up in conversation, usually prompted by his enquiry for my son Aran whom he had met and who was at boarding school in Newtown in Waterford. He sympathized with the homesickness of boarding school and with Aran being at 'a difficult age but tell me one that is not'. Sam added that we should heed the telling words: 'Nothing can be worse than this! Nothing – provided we can be sure that this is the worst.'

At a visit to Le Tiers Temps he was delighted to meet Tona again and he showed affection for my youngest son, Emmet, who had stood in for him in the photography for *The Beckett Country* as the boy on snow-clad Glencree and at the Forty Foot, where he refused to 'be a brave boy' and jump into the freezing water. My daughter Aphria's affection for the hedgehog in *Company* brought him back some eighty years and the reminiscence was not without pain. Tona and the children left after a short time and I stayed on talking and supping Irish whiskey with him.

Sam and I sometimes discussed the arts in Dublin and Ireland. I recounted how the smell of oranges in the Theatre Royal in Wexford during the performance of *Eritrea*, by bringing an olfactory dimension to the performance, had heightened my enjoyment. Sam was pleased to hear about the foundation of the National Concert Hall. He had been interviewed for the Joyce Centenary, which he thought was being done well. The story of Niall Sheridan going to see Joyce in Paris bearing a few pounds of Hafner's sausages and a bottle of Jameson amused him, and he was pleased that *Ulysses* was to be broadcast over twenty-four hours on Bloomsday. We joked over my suggestion in *The Irish Times* that Westmoreland Street should be renamed Boulevard Bloom.

Returning from a holiday in Venice I expounded on my love for the city. Sam recalled going there from Florence with Mario Esposito. He had been close to Bianca Esposito's sister, Vera, who lived outside Florence. Bianca taught him Italian in Ely Place, close to where George Moore had lived. He had heard her father play all the Beethoven sonatas, and though he was a competent pianist, he could not be compared to Arthur Rubenstein, whom he had listened to recently on television; there was only one word for his performance – 'magical!'

Mores were changing in Ireland, and I knew Sam would appreciate the story of my being invited by Aran's school in Newtown to speak to the sixth formers on *Waiting for Godot*, which was on the curriculum for the Leaving Certificate examination. During questions after my presentation, one of the girls asked my opinion on the recent controversial production of *Waiting for Godot* in Holland with a female cast, which Sam had contested legally without success. Not wishing to embarrass her by recounting Beckett's retort that 'women don't have prostates,' I meekly stated that Beckett was very clear on the gender of actors in all his plays. The student went on, however, to inform me that females could not play Vladimir and Estragon and she quoted the lines:

> Estragon: What about hanging ourselves?
> Vladimir: Hmm. It'd give us an erection.
> Estragon: (*highly excited*). An erection!
> Vladimir: With all that follows.
> Where it falls mandrakes grow.

She concluded by stating that it was not only ridiculous, but physiologically impossible, for Vladimir and Estragon to be played by females. Beckett was delighted that such freedom of expression was now possible in schools, adding that he could have done with her testimony in Amsterdam.

Sam read my books on subjects that I didn't think would interest him, and he did so with excruciating editorial diligence, much to my embarrassment. I sent him *The House of Industry Hospitals 1772–1987* in 1988, and when I visited him in Le Tiers Temps on rue Rémy-Dumoncel sometime later, on 1 February 1989, he gave me a piece of cardboard politely listing no fewer than ten spelling errors; the fact they were spread over the 300-page range showed he had read the entire book. His interest may have been kindled by the book being a history of the hospital where his schoolboy friend Alan Thompson had worked.

Sam always showed a genuine interest in my medical life, and a desire to understand my research work in hypertension. At one meeting I had come from Leiden, which he commented was an appropriate place for a doctor to have been. I elaborated on the medical history meeting I had attended and expressed disappointment that so little of the old university existed. He asked if Descartes had not spent time there, or was it Spinoza? We discussed Boerhaave and Einthoven.

He knew the former and I recounted Einthoven's Nobel-honoured creation of the electrocardiograph. I told him of my plan to go to Arcachon in search of Dominic Corrigan who had a street named after him in the town. Sam spent time there in the bad days in 1944. He remembered bathing and the pine forests coming down to the sea – the smell was pleasant, he said. He asked me about Corrigan and was amused at Joyce's reference to him in *Finnegans Wake* and was not too surprised by Corrigan's tussle with the Catholic hierarchy.

Sam also took interest in my hospital practice as a cardiologist, my difficulties with professional colleagues, particularly as an editor and journalist, and in my scientific pursuits. He was pleased when I told him a little sheepishly that he could now call me 'Professor'. His blue eyes lit up and smiling as only he could smile, he congratulated me warmly. But lest he be carried away, I hastened to add that the designation was merely a 'personal chair' and went on to explain that it was academic recognition of scientific achievement – it did not carry the administrative or teaching duties of a full professorship. 'Well, Eoin,' he responded, having taken a few moments to reflect on the pros and cons of this enlightenment, 'sounds to me more like a stool than a chair' and, warming to the analogy, he went on to reassure me that 'stools are much more useful than chairs, especially in bars where they allow the arse to be propped in propinquity to the elbow, the one balanced nicely in concert with the other so as to clutch the pint twixt counter and gob'. I have occupied three chairs, but none will be as dear to me as that first 'stool' – a warning never to take myself too seriously. I am grateful to Sam for this gentle awakening that has led me to view the nonsense of pomp and ceremony (with which my profession is obsessed) with a jaundiced eye.

Perhaps it was inevitable that Sam would enquire about human peculiarities that intrigued him. The heart and its control mechanism and its response to emotional stimuli were issues of curiosity. Indeed, I later discovered that he had figured out for himself a phenomenon that cardiologists had been slow to recognize. His hero Murphy was endowed with a remarkable physiological ability to voluntarily control his heart: 'Murphy had lately studied under a man in Cork called Neary. This man, at that time, could stop his heart more or less whenever he liked and keep it stopped, within reasonable limits, for as long as he liked.'

Sam was also fascinated by what he called the 'womb-tomb enigma'. We pondered if the reality of expulsion from the cosy womb into the misery of the world could influence the being who must inevitably face the vicissitudes of a hostile environment. Might the traumatic ejection itself not lead to anxieties and distressful symptoms in later life? The experience itself was unlikely to be remembered, but could the terror associated with the event not be stored subconsciously to cause anxiety when the fear was recalled in later life? In this regard Sam referred to his discussions with the psychoanalyst Wilfred Bion, whom he had attended in London in the early 1930s on the recommendation of Geoffrey Thompson.

Inevitably, Sam's declining health became a concern. His country retreat, which he described as 'a very modest place', was an escape from the burden of correspondence in Paris and he was pleased when he could manage there without having to use an oxygen cylinder. He worried that his car might also begin to decline but, to his surprise, it fired at first demand. The winter had done much damage to the plants, despite the efforts of his devoted helpers, man and wife, who looked after things for him. He worried about not being able to remain independent since he was unsteady when walking. The best time of the day was 7.30 pm when he had his Jameson.

Discussion in our later meetings was dominated by his increasing inability to write, his despair at being unable to create: 'Work finished, Eoin, nothing left.' He had just completed *Stirrings Still* and was pleased with Barbara Bray's suggestion for the title. He hoped that the special edition would provide financial assistance for Barney Rosset and John Calder. However, he yearned for inspiration for a final statement, 'the most exciting of all', but it seemed that he was waiting in vain to express 'nothingness'. He was alert to the possibility that a statement from the ruin that was now his mind might be an expression of 'senile infantilism'. He added that 'perhaps he had not decayed far enough'. He was depressed that no inspiration was forthcoming, even in the country where he drank up the silence and peace. The best he could do was 'Ochón agus Ochón! I'm dead but not gone.'

I suggested that the statement he wished for was unable to bypass the barriers he had erected for himself over the years and that only when they were sublimated could the voice escape to express itself. He agreed that there was nothing to do but wait, unless he called it a day, be 'sad and glad' to end it all, to write no more. We ended that discussion by agreeing that we both knew it was not yet time to blow the final whistle. But the threat of creative decline would not leave him. At another of our meetings, he lamented his inability to write and hoped 'it was not the end', that there might be a 'few drops to be wrung out yet' and he made the appropriate gesture of wringing a sponge. Sam was not willing to be forced into 'physical and cerebral immobility – frozen by it all – too easy to permit – must not let it happen – won't let it happen – not yet'. He was not prepared to succumb to a growing sense of cerebral impotence.

Edith Fournier entrusted me with memorabilia and some notes written by Beckett on scraps of paper. She wanted to destroy these but could not bring herself to do so and passed them on to me. Likewise, I found that these notes, which I shall call 'thoughts', had a tender beauty, which I believe should be preserved.[28] No doubt some worthy scholar might show that the nidus of a greater opus is among them. But even if they were just sparks destined to fall short of a fire, I find them beautiful as is, like tiny diamonds that could bedeck a piece of jewellery, but not having done so, are not diminished in their brilliance. I challenge those who criticize me for preserving the likes of the following snippets to say the world is the worse for my having done so:

Side 1.

Let go of my hand
(Pause. No louder)
Let go my hand.

Do you remember –
No. Yes or no.

Side 2.

Where are we now
now?
In the spare room.
Facing east.
It feels dark. Is
it night?
Not quite.
Twilight?
Yes. Twilight.
Sit me down on
the bed.
On the edge of the bed.
There is no bed.
No bed?
No bed.
What happened to the bed?

And a note: 'Vain entreaty spent all still. Pond still. The air. Not a breath. Dead still. The grass long grey. Self drooped once and for all. Ah once. Grass not the word. No word for that grass. That self. What next. All said. That said. Said and done. What's left. The light. Ah the light.'

My meetings made me realize that Sam's talent wasn't confined to his power of expression in prose, poetry and drama, but to his influence as a philosopher. Perhaps it is here that he holds hands so easily with a doctor in search of some meaning to the suffering of existence. There is a force in his writing that may not make one a better doctor but may at least awaken a realization of what suffering is about. Beckett shines a torch on existence with such accuracy that he has fulfilled the ambition made in youthful days of redefining the human condition within the confines of the 'tailpiece' that concludes *Watt*, 'the sum of the world's woes in nothingness enclose'.

I attempted to express my gratitude to my friend in *Hello, Sam* in 2011, closing my side of the dialogue with:

> Sam, you changed the way we see ourselves and those around us. I have been close to humanity in the doldrums, but I had not seen – had shut out the reality of suffering – until you showed me man unadorned: ugly, decrepit, depraved, laughing, despairing, but majestic in his nothingness and not always without hope. My dear friend, you gave me and so many others the courage to go on, and not only to go on, but to do so without being afraid to fail – the success, as it were, of failure was, in your philosophy, a matter of having the courage to dare to fail. In Paris, we used to part with you saying 'Make me a sign' – such was to be the signal for our next meeting. So now, Sam, I bid you farewell by asking that you 'Make me a sign.'[29]

In 1975, when Tona and I were in holiday in France, we became friends with Francis Evers. Francis was a forlorn presence in my life. He was a thin, hyperkinetic individual with a slight squint. He was sincere, scatter-brained, neurotic, exasperating, humourless but appreciative of the subtlety of humour. We shared a love of literature – one could say that he was obsessed with Beckett and his writing.

We met yearly and occasionally, when we had something to celebrate, dined at Le Procope on rue de l'Ancienne Comédie. On one of his early visits to Clifton Terrace, I mistakenly presumed that the plastic bag in his grasp carried gifts for the children but soon learned that this habitual accompaniment housed his precious supply of duty-free Gauloises or Marlboro cigarettes. His passionate love of conversation and chain-smoking could lead to conflagrations; my trousers and the skirt of a waitress at La Coupole being casualties at our first meeting.

Francis loved the intrigue of literary debate. Intellectual conversation was his métier. He would gladly stay up all night discussing literature, drama, controversial opinion on this or that writer but, most particularly, Beckett. We joined in a long-running and largely fruitless controversy in the correspondence columns of *The Irish Times* on the issue of copyright over the publication of Joyce's Trieste letters in 1976.

Francis knew Beckett for years but kept this relationship to himself. He also wrote critical essays on Beckett, but I cannot find any record of this. Beckett had sympathy for Francis's predicament, and I suspect gave him financial assistance from time to time. His friendship with Beckett is variously stated as being of such intimacy that they watched rugby international games between Ireland and France together, as is recorded by his anonymous obituarist.[30] In Dublin we visited graveyards searching for the resting place of Frank Beckett, and visited Beckett's childhood and adolescent homes, Cooldrinagh and New Place. These peregrinations provided the stuff of many midnight conversations, during which Francis never mentioned their close relationship.

Francis had many literary friends in Dublin. One of these was Ronnie Drew: he helped Drew survive many alcoholic jousts, with me providing medical support. One day Ronnie and I met by chance at Dublin Airport and, as he was telling me that he was on his way to Basel (I think) to be granted the freedom of the city or some such honour, we both became conscious of a tall figure circling around us. As we chatted on, the hovering enthusiast suddenly pounced on me, pencil and autograph book at the ready. I informed him that of the two bearded figures he had made the wrong choice and that I could not sing, which drew a rejoinder from Ronnie as he signed his autograph: 'For your information, neither can I!' Ronnie headed off to Switzerland, assuring me that he now had the content for his after-dinner speech that evening.

Francis was born in Dublin in the mid-1930s to a single mother in the days when such indiscretion was viewed with vicious societal rectitude. His childhood, which was spent in an orphanage and later in an industrial home, was extremely unhappy. Given the turbulent history of such institutions, it was inevitable that his unhappy youth left scars on his sensitive soul. However, he used his inherent love of literature to educate himself and to wrest himself from his deprived background. He left for England in the 1950s and did national service. He then went to Sydney, where he worked as a theatre critic and came to public prominence by defending the controversial design for the Sydney Opera House. He moved back from Australia to Paris, where he became correspondent for many other newspapers and news agencies, including *The Irish Times*, and made occasional broadcasts for RTÉ.

Francis established a fond relationship with Angeles Tomás, who managed a family pharmacy business in Villajoyosa, near Alicante, moving from Paris to Alicante in the 1980s to join Angeles, whom he referred to fondly as 'the girl'.

I visited Francis often at 29 rue Dauphine. He was writing what I presumed to be a novel. Evers regarded Beckett as a greater talent than Joyce because of 'the diversity of his expression – he can be seen as a novelist, a short-story writer, a poet and a dramatist, and moreover, as a philosopher – but then again, any writer worth his salt must philosophise at some point'. He urged me to write creatively and to forget history and science. Francis gave me his criticism of Beckett in the *Dublin Magazine* of 1958, which was impressive. Regrettably, none of his writings can be retrieved and those he gave me have not survived. Knowing that he had been working on a book, I wrote to Angeles after his death to see if it was extant in his papers, but she found nothing.

Evers suffered from gastric symptoms all his life and died in his sixties, probably from stomach cancer, on 19 December 1995. Many friends attended his memorial service in Clontarf. His anonymous obituarist summed up his enigmatic life by commenting that, although he had a unique network of friends, 'he was so discreet about them, that we ourselves did not realize we were part of a collective group of people from the arts, music and literature. He preserved his integrity in a way that is difficult in a city like Dublin.'

Barbara Bray and I became friends in the 1970s. She was excellent company and we enjoyed many evenings together in Paris, meeting in Les Deux Magots or the Café de Flore in Saint-Germain-des-Prés before discussing rather wild and far-fetched ideas into the small hours, often after too much wine liberated fantasies and dreams that would fade by dawn.[31] Our friendship and discussions rested on a common bond, a friendship, love and admiration for Samuel Beckett. As Beckett became terminally ill, my relationship with Barbara waned. Perhaps she expected too much from him or, put another way, attached excessive expectations to what had been an intimate intellectual and physical relationship.

Barbara had an astounding critical appreciation of literary endeavour and sought to expand my world by giving me books by Marguerite Duras, Jean Genet and Robert Pinget. She uplifted my doubt about *The Beckett Country* when she wrote in January 1987:

> My dear Eoin. The reason I haven't written much sooner about your marvellous book is that every page so moves me I am lost for words. What you have done for our beloved Sam and his work is worth whole libraries of exegesis and commentary. It is a monument to a monument. Little did I think I'd ever be grateful to anyone for producing another tome on this topic! But I do most sincerely add my thanks to all those other tributes you'll be receiving far into the future. Many congratulations. Overcome your modesty and be proud of yourself! Love Barbara.

Barbara occasionally shared her more intimate exchanges with Beckett. For example, how she – encouraging him when in the doldrums to write – mercilessly reminded him that the decline of ageing he was decrying should be seized upon as the challenge he had always espoused; the nothingness from which to fashion creativity. This provocative encouragement wasn't without effect. Beckett overcame the decline of age to write his remarkable last work, *Stirrings Still*, for which Barbara also proposed the title with humorous innuendo. Born from the nothingness of decline, *Stirrings Still* is (at least from the viewpoint of a physician) a magnificent testimony to creativity despite the decline of ageing.

Beckett's health was often raised in our meetings and correspondence. In keeping with the old-fashioned (and alas now often ignored) principle that what passes between a doctor and a patient is sacrosanct, I wrote to Barbara after his death, saying:

> I made a resolution when he died to respect his wish for total privacy concerning those last days – not because there was anything that might not be discussed – but rather because they were his moments. Also, there was (is) my professional role as a physician as well as a friend. I know you will understand.

During Sam's last illness I kept her informed of his progress. On one occasion she brought me a small carrier bag with a bottle of lime juice and some savouries, which she asked me to bring to him, and I took the package, though I knew he was in no condition to partake of the contents. There was an accompanying card: 'Dearest Sam. Just a word with all my love, as and for ever. Hope you feel better soon. I do understand everything ('There's love for you … Eh Joe!') I am sending a few odds and ends via kind Eoin, in hopes some may be useful. Grateful, reverent and loving thoughts every moment from Barbara.' When I returned to the Hôtel Balzac after a particularly long day at the hospital, during which I had had little to eat, I wolfed down the contents of the bag – but I had no sooner done so than I was assailed with memories of discussions with Barbara on the merits of euthanasia and the thought that she might have doctored either the lime juice or the savouries led to a restless night awaiting a fate with truly Beckettian overtones.

Barbara wrote to me after Beckett's death, signifying her intention to write a memoir: 'I've just agreed to write a short memoir about Sam. Not a biography, of course – a tribute to his goodness and greatness in terms of which he wouldn't disapprove, and which as far as I can see others are not quite likely to capture.' I replied: 'I wish your memoir well. I know you knew him so well that you would not do other then he would have wished.'

Stanley William (Bill) Hayter was a vivacious character who delighted in good conversation about literature and art. I recall a dinner party in Clifton Terrace at which he devised a scale to indicate the vibrancy of a particular blue. At the time of our friendship, I was unaware that his awards included a Commander of the Order of the British Empire (CBE), the Légion d'Honneur and Commander in the Ordre des Arts et des Lettres. On one occasion I asked Bill if he ever considered illustrating Beckett's work, as other artists had done, but he confided in me that he and Beckett had had a disagreement that prevented this being possible. He and his wife, Désirée, generously supported the Leventhal Scholarship, which has enabled many students to travel to Paris and elsewhere in the world to further their studies.

When I visited Hayter's Atelier 17 studio in Paris in 1984, I was unaware that Pablo Picasso, Alberto Giacometti, Joan Miró and Marc Chagall, among many other legendary artists, had studied printmaking there. The purpose of my visit was to accompany Hayter and Marion Leigh to a party to celebrate the recent success of an exhibition by the Peruvian painter Herman Braun-Vega in the Théâtre du Rond-Point.[32] When Marion and I arrived, Bill was perched precariously on a plank between two ladders spanning an enormous canvas onto which he was lavishing vibrantly coloured paint. The evening didn't get off to a good start when Marion asked what the painting represented. Bill muttered to me that if he damn well knew, he would not tell her. We eventually joined Désirée, Barbara Bray and John Montague at the party. Braun-Vega was well known for painting his artist friends and he had painted a fine portrait of Bill Hayter a year earlier. Much drink was consumed, and illicit affairs were in the making and near-consummation in the many alcoves and niches of the party-giver's house.

Con Leventhal introduced me to Avigdor Arikha who, with his wife Anne and their daughters Nola and Alba, entertained me in their flat on the Square du Pont Royal. Arikha had been deported from the Ukraine in 1941 to a labour camp and after studying art in Jerusalem, he settled in Paris, where he lived until his death in 2010. He and Beckett had been very close, but I found Arikha to be self-righteous and beyond friendship. Perhaps I was humbled by my inability to joust with him in art and art history on which he was an acknowledged authority. We did discuss Dublin and particularly Ethna MacCarthy, whom he had known and admired, and I sent him a copy of Seán O'Sullivan's portrait of her. Whatever our inability to establish an intellectual relationship may have been, I admired his painting, and on my visits to London I always called into the Redfern Gallery in London to see his latest work. At the time of my acquaintance with him in 1983, he had just painted an acclaimed portrait of the Queen Mother and I have notes from him on postcards illustrating this sensitive portrait. Marion Leigh gave me a set of four sketches of Con in a Parisian café by Avigdor, which are remarkable testimony to that period of his career during which he worked only in monocolour.

After Sam's death, Anne Atik published *How It Was: A Memoir of Samuel Beckett*, and her daughter Alba later published *Major/Minor* in which they reminisce (from different perspectives) on the many remarkable people, most notably Beckett (he was Alba's godfather), who formed the intellectual milieu in which they lived.[33] However, Anne Atik in her memoir of Beckett claims that a poem, 'Petit Sot', reproduced in an almost illegible facsimile that is not Beckett's handwriting, was the first poem Beckett wrote. In fact, there is irrefutable evidence from Edith Fournier and Jérôme Linden, who had the proofs, that the poem was written by his wife Suzanne, and this travesty of fact, understandably and rightly, has led to a heated rebuttal; the debacle was recounted by Gerry Dukes in his review of *How It Was* for *The Independent* in 2012.[34]

I only knew Jérôme Linden and his wife, Annette, as distant figures, but we met frequently during Becket's last illness. Jérôme was one of the sincerest people I have ever had the pleasure of knowing and his loyalty to Beckett was absolute. He had accepted the Nobel Prize on Beckett's behalf in 1969 and throughout his life remained one of his closest confidants. Linden's death, in 2001, was an event of national importance in France.[35]

Acknowledgments

What's left. The light. Ah the light!

This memoir has been in gestation for some years and many people have assisted me in compiling a final text. Inevitably, I will omit to pay gratitude to some of those who assisted me, or I will fail to convey the magnitude of support from others. I can only crave forgiveness for any such shortcomings.

This memoir focuses on my life as a doctor in active clinical practice and I have not included the many activities that I have become involved with in retirement; these have involved research and administrative projects with the Irish Heart Foundation, the Irish Skin Foundation, the International Society of Hypertension and the European Society of Hypertension and collaborating with Alan Gilsenan in the making of his evocative *Ghosts of Baggotonia*.

The earliest drafts of the memoir were read by Edith Fournier and the present structure owes much to her helpful criticism. Gerald Dawe has given generously of his time to guide me in editing the early drafts, and he has kept a close watch on the development of the text. It is fair to say that the memoir would not have reached publication were it not for his support.

My former colleague, and lifelong friend, Dato Dr Leslie Lam, who has achieved international renown for his innovative contributions to cardiology in Singapore, has provided financial support and enthusiasm over many years for the creation and maintenance of the O'Brien/Lam Collection in the James Joyce Library of University College Dublin. I acknowledge with gratitude my use of the valuable archives in this collection.

John Banville, who can do with words what Mozart did with chords, encouraged me to persist with the memoir despite many moments of despondency. I am most grateful to him for writing a foreword in which he touches poignantly on revelatory moments in my past.

Robert Ballagh, who gave so generously of his time and expertise in illustrating *The Beckett Country; Samuel Beckett's Ireland* in 1986, has remained a close friend and we indulge often in reminiscences of a past Dublin we shared. He has been a constant source of encouragement and a further bond was established recently when he was commissioned to paint my portrait for University College Dublin.

Desmond Morris, who appreciated the surrealistic inclinations of Nevill Johnson which dominated much of my friendship with the artist, kindly agreed to endorse the memoir.

I am greatly indebted to Jonathan Williams, who suggested many modifications and painstakingly made grammatical corrections to the entire text.

I am grateful to Brendan Lynch for allowing me to quote from his many books on literary Dublin.

I needed detail and assurance on a variety of past associations and events and I am grateful for helpful responses from Stella Aillaud, Edward Beckett, Raymond Bell, Alan Gilsenan, Dickon Hall, Helen Hamlyn, Galway Johnson, Cecily Kelleher, Colum Kenny, Pat and Paul Kenny, Hugh Kerins, John Loughman, Francis Lynch, Pierce Meagher, John Minihan, Brenda Moore-McCann, Barbara Novak, Ted and Ursula O'Brien, Mary O'Doherty, Seamus O'Mahony, David Owen, Frank Powell, Vera Skrabanek, Kieran Taaffe, Adam Tattersall, Marcus Thompson, Gerald Tomkin, Maura West, Andrew Woolfson, Peter Woolfson. My thanks to members of my family, who provided many helpful details: Róisín Buree, Ronan Lyons, Aphria O'Brien, Berna O'Brien, Marie-Josephine O'Brien, Niall O'Brien, Tona O'Brien, Eda Sagarra, Geraldine O'Brien and Bosie Wallgren. Rosemary Byrne gave me diligent secretarial assistance.

I addressed medical queries to, and received helpful responses from, Garret Beevers, David Bouchier-Hayes, Eamon Dolan, Desmond Fitzgerald, Garret FitzGerald, Simon Lyons, Neil Poulter, Jan Staessen, George Stergiou and Joseph Walshe.

I would like to thank Dr Aidan Collins, whose knowledge of Ireland's medical and literary history prompted many helpful suggestions.

The team at Lilliput Press showed remarkable patience in complying with my many demands. My sincere thanks to Antony Farrell, Djinn von Noorden, Jennifer Brady, Ruth Hallinan and all the staff at Lilliput who have prepared the manuscript for publication.

It seems appropriate to devote some attention to the many people whose presence created the ambience out of which the memoir arose, or put another way, to mention the people around me who attracted me away from medicine to literature and art. Seamus and Marie Heaney touched my life on many occasions. Tom Flanagan came to see me whenever he was in Dublin. Tony Cronin was always available for advice, and I provided him with information for his biographical work *Samuel Beckett: The Last Modernist*. Christy Cahill, who had been Ben Kiely's literary protégé and who later became editor of *The Recorder* on which I was an editorial board member with

Seamus Heaney and Brian O'Doherty, among others, for many years, continues to share his literary ambitions with me. Poor Philip Casey, who so stoically suffered much during life only to be snatched away prematurely by cancer before he could complete his literary work, which he was so willing to share with others. Michael Colgan, director par excellence, who shared my enthusiasm for the work of Samuel Beckett and Barry McGovern, who not only gave Beckett's drama a unique Irish presence but who also sought to explore the essence that inspired his work. Gerry Dukes has helped me with many literary endeavours and, together with Brid, we have shared literary and artistic occasions together. Terry Byrne, a talented actor and producer of amateur drama, has been a friend for many years and he persuaded Aer Lingus to support the *Beckett Country Exhibition*. David Davison, whose photography is indispensable to many of my books, especially *The Beckett Country*, in which he portrayed landscape and architecture with sensitivity. Leo Cullen, a gentle writer, with whom I shared many conversations as we swam in the soothing waters of Seapoint. Harry Crosbie, a man of ideas who, supported by his ebullient wife, Rita, has never been afraid to dare to fail. Richard Lewis, master of femininity in haute couture, together with his partner, Jim, was an ever-present figure of cultural sensitivity. Maeve Binchy, with whom I shared many reminiscences about our common schooldays and had the audacity to suggest to her that she should try to write serious rather than frivolous nonsense. Seán Ó Mórdha, whose films on Joyce and Beckett are expressions of beauty dependent on cinematic skill and careful research, often discussed with me his enlightened optimism for television, which alas was not shared by his superiors. Trevor West, one of the finest mathematical minds to grace the academic portals of Trinity College, who also contributed so selflessly to the sporting life of the university, and whose wife, Maura, was a lifelong friend to my wife, Tona, and bridesmaid at our wedding, was a frequent presence both in Dublin and when we enjoyed the warm hospitality of the family home in Midleton, Co. Cork.

When I ponder what it was that attracted me to the arts, I must acknowledge family influences, particularly my father and my maternal grandmother, but I think also that childhood and student days immersed in a little patch of territory that can now be topographically designated as Baggotonia, and the artistic movement it nurtured may have alerted me, however subconsciously, to the richness of creative endeavour that surrounded me. Without Tona's support, encouragement, and advice, my past would have been devoid of content. My children, Aran, Emmet and Aphria, who all had the privilege of meeting Sam Beckett, supported me in my efforts to preserve the memory of times past, and at times were active participants in my reminiscences; for example, my son Emmet stood in for the young Beckett in many photographs and, my daughter, Aphria, acted as courier to transport the proofs of *The Beckett Country* from Dublin to Cork.

Endnotes

1. FAMILY ORIGINS

1. About 75 per cent of the RIC were Roman Catholic and about 25 per cent were of various Protestant denominations. The 1921 Anglo-Irish Treaty disbanded the RIC, which was replaced by the Garda Síochána in the Irish Free State and the Royal Ulster Constabulary in Northern Ireland. RIC salaries were low, on the assumption that milk, eggs, butter and potatoes would be provided as gifts from local people. Constables in charge of police stations were required to make regular reports to their superiors and were moved frequently to prevent the development of close acquaintanceships. A constable was not permitted to marry until he had been in the force for some years and would not be drafted to serve in his or his wife's home county.

2. Clonmellon has a modest claim on history. An obelisk marks the position where Sir Walter Raleigh planted some of the first potatoes he imported to Ireland, and the occasion is celebrated by an annual Potato Festival.

3. William (known as Willie) was born in 1895 in Ballinrobe; John (known as Jack) was born in 1896 in Waterford; Mary Josephine (known as Mai) was born in 1898 in Waterford; Thomas Joseph was born and died in 1899 in Tubbercurry; Eveleen was born in 1901 in Tubbercurry, County Sligo; Gerard Thomas (my father) was born in 1906 in Thurles.

4. A newspaper cutting from *The Glasgow Observer* on 12 September 1925 gives a lengthy account of the career of Dr Eveleen O'Brien, 'Distinguished Irish Graduate, Catholic Lady Doctor'.

5. Michael Viney is an artist, author, broadcaster and journalist. He was born in Brighton, England, in 1933. He is best known for his writings on nature.

6. E. Sagarra, *Envoy Extraordinary: Professor Smiddy of Cork* (Institute of Public Administration, 2018).

7. Pearl Anna Maria (1903–2003) trained as a physiotherapist and masseuse. She had a relationship with a Spanish count in Washington, culminating in a bigamous marriage that was eventually annulled. She later married an English orthopaedic surgeon, Charles Louis, and they had two children, Roisín and Charles. She died in England in 2003. Cecilia Maria (1904–1994) married Kevin Roantree O'Shiel, an Irish politician, barrister and civil servant who devoted much of his time to championing Irish Home Rule. A biography, *Kevin O'Shiel: Tyrone Nationalist and Irish State-Builder*, written by his daughter, Eda Sagarra, was published

in 2013. Muriel (my mother) (1907–1984) graduated with distinction as a medical doctor from the RCSI and married my father, Gerard T. O'Brien. Ita (1910–2002) was a radiologist who married Dr Harry O'Flanagan. Ethna (1918–2003) married Dr J. McSorley. The only son, Sarsfield (1905–1978), emigrated to the United States and worked in the motor industry business.

8. The approach taken by Smiddy in his addresses to influential bodies is apparent in 'The Economic Conditions and Policies of the Irish Free State', an address by his Excellency the Right Honourable Timothy A. Smiddy before the Empire Club of Canada, Toronto, 15 April 1926.

9. M. Kennedy. 'Smiddy, Timothy Aloysius'. *Dictionary of Irish Biography.* October 2009.

10. J.A. Gaughan, *Alfred O'Rahilly* (Kingdom Books, 1986). As a schoolboy I was sent to 'assist' O'Rahilly, who was residing in Blackrock College where he was compiling his tome, *The Life of Christ.*

11. The family attribution for this portrait is that it was a copy portrait of *Ball, the astronomer* by Rembrandt. I am grateful to John Loughman who ascertained that the painting is a copy of a portrait in the Musée du Louvre by Ferdinand Bol of an unknown mathematician, signed and dated 1658. Bol was a pupil of Rembrandt's in the late 1630s and his work has been confused with that of his teacher. The Musée du Louvre allows a limited number of copyists, both amateurs and professionals, access to a single painting each year under strict conditions, a practice that dates from the late eighteenth century.

12. *Systematic Case-taking: A Practical Guide to the Examination and Recording of Medical Cases for the Use of Medical Students* was written by Henry Lawrence McKisack, physician to the Royal Victoria Hospital in Belfast and published in London in 1912. My father's copy is inscribed by McKisack to Dr Jock O'Carroll, a senior member of the staff of the Richmond Hospital from 1886 to 1931, who presumably gave it to my father when he joined the staff in 1932.

13. Sir Peter Kerley (1900–78) was a radiologist from Dundalk, Ireland, and a graduate of UCD. A reference reads: 'Dr. Gerard O'Brien attended my department in the Royal Chest Hospital, London, from November 1934 until April 1935. He also took the course for the Cambridge Diploma in Radiology during the same period. He is a keen and able worker, and I have a deep admiration for his profound knowledge of diseases of the heart and lungs.'

14. G.T. O'Brien. 'Some Chronic Non-Tuberculous Pulmonary Conditions', *Ir J Med Sci*, 1937;12.10. 617–25.

15. G.T. O'Brien. 'Three Irish Pioneers of Medicine'. *Ir J Med Sci*, 1949;1–11.

16. H. Counihan. Obituary: Dr Gerard Thomas O'Brien. FRCPI, *J Ir Med Ass*, 1973; 66:145.

17. *The Irish Times* 7 December 1934 and press cutting. Operation on a boy. Surgeon sued in Dublin. Unusual Case; Press cuttings November 1934. The Smiddy Archive in the O'Brien/Lam Collection. Special Collections. The James Joyce Library. University College Dublin.

2. CHILDHOOD

1. A. O'Keeffe, 'The day Dev said sorry over suicide of the world's worst war criminal'. *The Herald*, 30 April 2015. This article notes that 'as news of the evil dictator's demise reached

Dublin, then Taoiseach of neutral Ireland, Éamon de Valera, made a controversial visit to offer condolences to the ambassador Eduard Hempel. The swastika flag flew at half-mast at the red brick house on Dublin's Northumberland Road, but few people mourned the loss of one of the 20th Century's most vile leaders.'

2.   T. Murphy (Director of Dublin Zoo from 1957 to 1984), *Some of My Best Friends Are Animals* (Paddington Press, 1979).

3.   Paul and Pat Kenny, sons of Sarah's keeper, have confirmed that my father's tale as related by him to me is true in so far as Sarah escaped from her pound and took cover in the lake, but my father may have wandered from the path of truth to embellish the tale.

4.   E. O'Brien, *A Century of Service: The City of Dublin Skin and Cancer Hospital 1911–2011* (Anniversary Press, Dublin, 2011).

5.   E. Kinsella, *Leopardstown Park Hospital 1917–2017: A Home for Wounded Soldiers*, (Leopardstown Park Hospital, 2017).

6.   A.F. Carthy, *The Treatment of Tuberculosis in Ireland from the 1890s to the 1970s: A Case Study of Medical Care in Leinster* (Thesis for the degree of PhD Department of History, National University of Ireland Maynooth, 2015), p. 311.

7.   E. O'Brien, L. Browne, K. O'Malley (eds), *The House of Industry Hospitals 1772–1987: The Richmond, Whitworth and Hardwicke (St. Laurence's Hospital). A Closing Memoir* (Anniversary Press, Dublin, 1988).

8.   These patients were given a bed in different wards where they were available for teaching clinics.

9.   N. Lomb, O'Connell, Daniel Joseph Kelly (1896–1982)'. *Australian Dictionary of Biography*, Vol. 18, 2012. Daniel O'Connell achieved considerable astronomical stature for giving scientific credibility to the Green Flash phenomenon when he published *The Green Flash and Other Low Sun Phenomena* (in 1958). At the Vatican Observatory O'Connell installed the observatory's largest instrument, a 60/90-cm Schmidt telescope. He had personal friendships with three popes and was especially close to Pope Pius XII. In 1970, O'Connell, retired from his observatory post but continued as president (1968–72) of the Pontifical Academy of Sciences.

10.   John Charles McQuaid (1895–1973), was the Catholic Primate of Ireland and Archbishop of Dublin between December 1940 and January 1972. He was known for the unusual amount of influence he had over successive governments, especially on issues relating to sexuality and contraception. He is the subject of many biographies, such as: John Cooney, *John Charles McQuaid: Ruler of Catholic Ireland* (O'Brien Press Ltd., 2009).

11.   St Conleth's School is named after Conleth, a sixth-century Irish monk who was a moulder of precious metals.

12.   Denis Donoghue and I had no communication with each other for some sixty years. I wrote to Denis in 2016 asking if he remembered this brief and inconsequential moment in his life. He responded: 'Dear Eoin: I remember you, your parents, your home, but virtually nothing else that would be of any use to you in your memoir. Specifically, I have no recollection of my arm in a sling or any fall that would have necessitated it. That indicates the feebleness of my memory at age 87. I wish you well and would like to read the memoir …' (5 April 2016).

13.	Dara Ó Lochlainn and I were good friends at St Conleth's and having both been dismissed from there to Castleknock College for having offended Catholic propriety, the friendship became even stronger. Dara, who was a talented artist and jazz musician, died on 20 December 1992 at Harold's Cross Hospice, Dublin, after suffering from throat cancer for seven years.

John Gilmartin was the most precocious member of my class at St Conleth's. He cut salacious snippets on sex and gynaecology from his father's *Medical Encyclopaedia* that were never missed because his father, Tommy, an anaesthetist, would presumably not have had interest in this section. Most of his life was spent in the company of his parents and their friends at 32 Lower Baggot Street. His obituarist, Charles Lysaght, aptly states: 'His parents' world rather than that of his contemporaries fashioned his outlook.' He was a devout Catholic and, thinking he had a vocation for the priesthood, entered, as might be expected, the fashionable order of the Birmingham and Brompton Oratories. He died on 19 July 2019, aged eighty. See: 'Charles Lysaght. Appreciation'. John Gilmartin. *The Irish Times*, 9 December 2019.

14.	From Psalms xx 7. '*Hi in curribus et hi in equis; nos autem in nomine Domini Dei nostri invocabimus.*' ('Some trust in chariots or horses; we, however, [trust] in the Name of the Lord.') The College ethos was: 'To have a College which is concerned with the development of the Whole person in a Christian atmosphere Which encourages involvement in a balance of Religious, Intellectual, Cultural and Sporting Activities And which promotes the growth of Self-worth and Respect for Others In the spirit of St Vincent de Paul.' See: J. Murphy, *Nos Autem: Castleknock College and Its Contribution* (Gill & Macmillan,1996).

15.	I 'borrowed' two books for myself, which I still have: a leather-bound gilded copy of *The Poetical Works of Lord Byron*, published by Oxford University Press in 1923 and a 1918 Oxford edition of the *Poetical Works of William Wordsworth*.

3. THE STUDY OF MEDICINE

1.	D. Fallon, 'From McDaid's to Grogan's: The Legendary Paddy O'Brien', Come Here to Me! Dublin Life and Culture (website), 1 May 2018.

2.	A. Norman Jeffares, 'The Hay Hotel', *The Poems & Plays of Oliver St John Gogarty* (Colin Smyth Ltd. 2001), p. 454.

3.	'The Ireland That We Dreamed Of', 1943. *Éamon de Valera (1882–1975)*. RTÉ archives, 17 March 1943.

4.	J. Banville, *Time Pieces: A Dublin Memoir* (Hachette Books Ireland, 2016), p. 103.

5.	Kevin Duffy returned from the Royal Navy to become a successful and much-esteemed GP in Daingean, County Offaly. He died from a stroke in August 2007.

6.	Tom McDonald and I were both offered fellowships at the Mayo Clinic but whereas I dismissed the option because of the likelihood of being drafted to serve in Vietnam, McDonald took the opposite course. He served with distinction in Vietnam and was decorated for bravery. He joined the staff of the Mayo Clinic as a consultant in the Department of Otorhinolaryngology (head and neck surgery) and was later was appointed Chair of the Department and Vice-Chairman of the Mayo Clinic's Board of Governors. In 1990 he was made an Honorary

Fellow of his alma mater, the RCSI. He died in September 2019 at the age of seventy-nine. A memoir entitled *Far from Ballynahinch* by Thomas McDonald and Michael Ransom is due to be published in 2023.

7. John Lynch, after spending a few years in the army medical corps in Germany and working as a GP in the UK, specialized in psychiatry, which he practised in Clonmel. He died at his home in Clonmel on 17 March 2004 aged sixty-eight.

8. Lyn Nash was not long for this life. Depressed and overcome by alcohol, he shot himself in a field in Oxfordshire on 20 May 1978 at the age of forty years. My obituary for the *BMJ*, which was declined, concluded: 'Then as illness took its hold, he saw very clearly the indignity of the future.'

9. Tommy Bouchier-Hayes joined the British army halfway through his medical studentship and, after serving his time after qualification, decided to make a career in Her Majesty's Service. He achieved the rank of major and became professor of general practice at the Royal Army Medical College, Millbank, and in this capacity co-authored several popular books on examination technique and emergencies in general practice. He died in London from atherosclerosis on 13 September 2002, aged sixty-five. R.P. Craig, in an obituary in the *BMJ*, wrote that Bouchier-Hayes 'was as near to an anarchist as the British Army could ever possibly tolerate.' *BMJ* 2003;326:603.

10. E. O'Brien. 'Obituary. John David Henry Widdess (1906–1982)'. *Ir Med J*, 1982;75:263.

11. J.D. Garry, *A Dublin Anatomist: Tom Garry* 1884–1963 (Black Cat Press, 1984).

12. As a student I was taught first to take a history, then to proceed to examination and finally propose a diagnosis. When I became a teacher I advocated changing the order of clinical assessment by taking a history but then making a provisional diagnosis before proceeding to examine the patient. E. O'Brien. 'History, Diagnosis and Then Examination'. *Ir Med J*, 1979;72:499.

13. E. Smith, M. Delargy. 'Locked-in Syndrome'. *BMJ* 2005;330:406–9. Reference to the 'locked-in syndrome' may be found also in the writings of Alexandre Dumas and Émile Zola, in the characters of Noirtier de Villefort and Madame Raquin.

14. The eponym Sydenham is attached to the condition in recognition of the British physician Thomas Sydenham (1624–1689) who first described it. The alternate eponym, 'Saint Vitus' Dance', refers to Saint Vitus, a Christian saint who was persecuted by Roman emperors and died as a martyr in AD 303.

15. W. Stokes, *A Treatise on the Use of the Stethoscope* (Edinburgh, 1825). This was the first publication in English attesting to the beneficial use of the stethoscope.

16. 'On 1 April 1832 Dr D.J. Corrigan published a paper entitled 'On Permanent Patency of the Mouth of the Aorta, or Inadequacy of the Aortic Valve' in the *Edinburgh Medical and Surgical Journal*, 1832. In the Clinique Médicale de l'Hôtel Dieu de Paris, the celebrated physician Armand Trousseau taught his students the clinical manifestations of the '*maladie de Corrigan*' and the Corrigan eponym was first used in print in *La Lancette Française: Gazette Des Hopitaux* in 1838.
See also E. O'Brien, *Conscience and Conflict: A Biography of Sir Dominic Corrigan, 1802–1880* (Glendale Press, Dublin 1983).

17. A water-hammer toy was made by sealing water in a vacuum in a glass tube, which when shaken gave a peculiar knocking sound.

18. Southey's uncle was one of the 'Lake Poets' with William Wordsworth and Samuel Taylor Coleridge. Southey was a lifelong friend of Charles Lutwidge Dodgson (Lewis Carroll).

19. I donated my father's device to the Arthur Hollman Collection of The British Cardiovascular Society, 9 Fitzroy Square, London.

20. Before the founding of The Rotunda Hospital, the pregnant women among the populous poor of Dublin were completely without medical care. The founder of the first lying-in hospital, Bartholomew Mosse, was a doctor of remarkable compassion and energy, who devoted his life to erecting a hospital for these unfortunate women. He raised money through lotteries, concerts and entertainments to enable him to build not only the first such hospital but also one of considerable architectural beauty. The hospital was granted a charter and opened in 1745 with Mosse as the first Master. Unfortunately, he did not live long to direct the hospital, which survives as a lasting tribute to a remarkable humanist.

21. E. O'Brien, G. Dawe (eds), *Ethna MacCarthy: Poems* (The Lilliput Press, 2019), p. 30.

4. A JOURNEY TO SPECIALIZATION

1. E. O'Brien, L. Browne, K. O'Malley (eds), *The Richmond, Whitworth and Hardwicke (St Laurence's Hospital): A Closing Memoir* (Anniversary Press. Dublin, 1988), pp. 107–9.

2. As house surgeon, my main commitment was to Paddy Carey, but I also worked with the neurosurgeons Johnny Lanigan and Sandy Pate.

3. McConnell published nine papers in distinguished international journals, which attests to a considerable scientific achievement. J.C. Duddy, B. Kennerk. 'Adams Andrew McConnell (1884–1972): Pioneer of Irish Neurosurgery'. *Brit J Neurosurg*, 2015;29:1, 4–8.

4. The procedure became obsolete when levodopa proved so beneficial in the 1960s, a drug immortalized by Oliver Sacks in his book *Awakenings*. Many years later I had the opportunity of recounting the lack of scientific evidence for stereotactic procedures with Sacks over dinner in my home with my wife and Paul Hamlyn. While Sacks was a remarkable writer, I found him to be an unpleasant person.

5. M. Coleman, 'P. Murray' *Dictionary of Irish Biography*, October 2009. Murray had an outstanding rugby career. His son John Brendan, also a doctor, who worked with me in the Richmond Hospital, won an international rugby cap against France in 1964.

6. Eugene O'Connor became a successful GP who practised for many decades in the inner city of Dublin. He died on 8 February 2015.

7. Cherry Orchard Fever Hospital opened in the 1950s to replace the old Cork Street Fever Hospital, which had served in the densely populated Liberties since 1804. It consisted of eleven ward blocks on a 74-acre site, one of which was the Regional Polio Centre. The need for fever hospitals would decline in the next few decades with the eradication of many common infectious diseases, such as measles, tuberculosis, smallpox, diphtheria and poliomyelitis. Cherry Orchard closed as a hospital for infectious diseases in 2002. See F. Brady. *Cherry Orchard Hospital Archive*, Royal College of Physicians of Ireland Heritage Centre. 2015.

8.	The claustrophobic horror of being incarcerated in an iron lung is depicted in the novel by J.G. Farrell, *The Lung* (Hutchinson & Co. Ltd., 1965).

	The story of the last survivor from Cherry Orchard, Peter Costello, has been the subject of the TV documentary *Would You Believe: Iron Will. 'The man in the iron lung'*. The longest survivor in an iron lung was the remarkable writer Martha Mason, who came first in her class when she studied for a BA in English from Wake Forest University, North Carolina. The Salk vaccine in the late 1950s brought polio under control and eliminated the disease in industrialized countries.

9.	The laboratory was dependent on philanthropic funding. Social events organized by Jack Cruise in the Olympia Theatre and Ben Dunne, the founder of Dunnes Stores, were regular occurrences. The laboratory was renamed the Colman K. Byrnes Research Centre in 1970. 'Douglas Thornes. 'Appreciation. Oncologist with a Belief in the Power of Intuition', *The Irish Times*, 27 March 2004.

10.	E. O'Brien, R.D. Thornes, D. O'Brien, B. Hogan. 'Inhibition of Antiplasmin and Fibrinolytic Effect of Protease in Patients with Cancer', *Lancet*, 1968;1:173–6; Anon. 'Protease and Cancer', *Lancet*, 1968; i:198.

11.	Founded originally as a workhouse in 1733, an infirmary was later provided that became Dudley Road Hospital in 1887. See G.W. Hearn, 'Dudley Road Hospital 1887–1987' (Postgraduate Centre, Dudley Road Hospital, 1987). The hospital would later be renamed The Birmingham City Hospital.

12.	Other consultants I worked for included: Ron Fletcher, an endocrinologist who had written a popular book, *Lecture Notes on Endocrinology*; Brian McConkey, a rheumatologist, who impressed me with his reliance on data to assess disease progress. Michael Small was a superb clinical neurologist, but he did not publish any significant papers.

13.	Paton had been trained in the Hammersmith Hospital by Sheila Sherlock, the international doyen of liver disease. One obituarist may be correct in criticizing Paton for lack of imagination and inadequate ambition, but he possessed a very fine intellect that brought him into conflict with the obduracy of the administrative ranks of the profession. C. Richmond. Alex Paton Obituary. *The Guardian*, 27 September 2015.

14.	The Royal College of Physicians of London was founded in 1518 by Royal Charter from King Henry VIII. It wasn't easy for me to gain acceptance to sit this exam. With a Licentiate from RCSI and not a degree, I was barred from sitting the membership exam of the English colleges and from eligibility for doctorate degrees in any university. However, the consultants in Dudley Road Hospital, who were themselves fellows of the London College, supported an application for special consideration on my behalf, and I was granted permission to sit the membership exam.

15.	E. O'Brien. 'Personal View'. *BMJ*, 1972;3:230.

16.	During his career as a cardiologist, John Mackinnon went diligently about his work without seeking attention. So too his passing attracted little comment. See: RCP Editor. John Mackinnon. *Munks Roll*. 1922–2016. Vol XII.

	The other members of the Cardiac Department were Shyam Singh, a somewhat irascible Indian cardiologist, grandson of the last Maharajah of Ajaigarh, who was innovative in developing cardiac catheterisation in children and David Eddy was Senior Registrar. The ECG department was run by the kindly and efficient Jill Plant.

17. D.G. Julian. 'The History of Coronary Care Units'. *Br Heart J*, 1987;57:497–502.

18. J.R. Jude. 'Personal Reminiscences of the Origin and History of Cardiopulmonary Resuscitation (CPR)'. *Am J Cardiol*, 2003;92:956–63.

19. S.P. Abhilash, N. Namboodiri. 'Sudden Cardiac Death: Historical Perspectives'. *Ind Heart J*, 2014;66:S4–9.

20. R. Adams. 'Cases of Diseases of the Heart, Accompanied with Pathological Observations'. *Dublin Hospital Reports*, 1827;4:353–453.
W. Stokes. 'Observations on Some Cases of Permanently Slow Pulse'. *Dublin Quarterly Journal of Medicine*, 1846;2:73–85.

21. Y. Pilcher, M.K. Healy. 'The Birmingham (Lucas) Pacemaker: A Follow-up with Particular Reference to Dependence and Parasystole'. *Brit Heart J*, 1972;34:1052–56.

22. J.D. Eddy, E.T. O'Brien, S.P. Singh. 'Glucagon and Haemodynamics of Acute Myocardial Infarction'. *BMJ*, 1969;4:663–5.

23. M.H. Pappworth. *Human Guinea Pigs: Experimentation on Man* (Routledge, 1967). This book became a sensation that was debated on television, in the media and in parliament, and predictably it outraged academic physicians who were then able to experiment on patients with impunity. Pappworth's book was a major influence in the establishment of ethics committees to supervise clinical research, and in the introduction of medical ethics as an academic discipline. It was not surprising that this outspoken physician was not held in high regard by the establishment of medicine, to which honest criticism was anathema. The Royal College of Physicians in London waited fifty-seven years before awarding him the honour of a fellowship, which it did in 1994, one year before his death. His obituarist, Christopher Booth, wrote: 'There have always been those who have been regarded as pestilential nuisances by their more conventional colleagues. Thomas Wakley, the first editor of *The Lancet*, was one. Maurice Pappworth was undoubtedly another. Yet, like Wakley, he was responsible for doing more by his vehement campaigning for patients' interests than anyone of his time in Britain.'
I wrote a review for Pappworth's popular aide-mémoire for medical students and membership examination candidates: E.T. O'Brien. 'Review: A Primer of Medicine by M.H. Pappworth'. *BMJ*, 1971;577:486.
His daughter has written a biography of her father: J. Seldon, *The Whistle-Blower: The Life of Maurice Pappworth* (University of Buckingham Press, 2018).

24. E. O'Brien. 'Cardiac Biopsy'. *BMJ*, 1972;2:420.

25. E. O'Brien, *Seapoint, Sea, Sky and Spires* (Anniversary Press, 2017).

26. E. O'Brien, *The Weight of Compassion & Other Essays* (The Lilliput Press, 2012), p. 158.

27. D. Smith, *Dissecting Room Ballads* (Black Cat Press, 1984), p. 16.

28. A. Norman Jeffares (ed.), 'Ringsend (After Reading Tolstoi)', *The Poems & Plays of Oliver St John Gogarty* (Colin Smyth Ltd., 2001), p.111.

29. E. O'Brien. 'Lunch at Ealing Abbey: A Memory of Dom Peter Flood', *Ir Med J*, 1979;72: 40–1.

30. The Charitable Infirmary, which opened in 1718, was followed by Dr Steevens' Hospital in 1733, Mercer's Hospital in 1734, the Rotunda Lying-In Hospital in 1745, the Meath Hospital and Sir Patrick Dun's Hospital in 1792, to name just five of many that sought to alleviate the intolerable state of the sick and poor of the city.

31. E. O'Brien, *Messiah: An Oratorio by George Frideric Handel* (The Black Cat Press, 1986).

32. Leslie Lam. Wikipedia, 29 November 2021. Many years later he would assist me in cataloguing my papers for deposition in the O'Brien/Lam Collection in the James Joyce Library of University College Dublin. Lam was to the forefront of introducing new cardiological technologies to Singapore, which are likely to have worldwide application.

33. E. O'Brien. 'A Case for Renaming Beaumont Hospital', *Ir Med Times*, 9 February 2018, p. 14.

5. THE WIDER WORLD OF MEDICINE

1. E.T. O'Brien, J. MacKinnon, 'Propranolol and Polythiazide in Treatment of Hypertension'. *Br Heart J* 34 (1972), pp. 1042–4.
   E. O'Brien, 'Beta-Blockers in the Treatment of Hypertension'. *J Ir Med Ass*, 1973;66:222.

2. E. O'Brien, 'Hypertension – Its Nature and Treatment'. *J Ir Coll Phys & Surg*, 1975;4:108.

3. On this journey I reminded myself of George Pickering's scathing opinion of research doctors: 'Essential hypertension is a type of disease not hitherto recognised in medicine, in which the defect is quantitative not qualitative. It is difficult for doctors to understand because it is a departure from the ordinary process of binary thought to which they were brought up. Medicine in its present state can count to 2 but not beyond.' G. Pickering, *High Blood Pressure* (Churchill Livingstone, 1968), p. 600.
   I would later become a close friend of Pickering's son, Tom, who carried forward his father's remarkable scientific reputation in hypertension, and, it might be argued, surpassed him. I gave the first Thomas Pickering Memorial Lecture in New York after Tom's all too early death in 2009. E. O'Brien First Thomas Pickering Memorial Lecture: 'Ambulatory Blood Pressure Measurement is Essential for the Management of Hypertension'. *J Clin Hyperten*, 2012;12:836–47.

4. The stimulus for the Framingham initiative had been the sudden death of Franklin D. Roosevelt from hypertension, heart failure and stroke in 1945. S.S. Mahmood, D. Levy, R.S. Vasan, T.J. Wang. 'The Framingham Heart Study and the Epidemiology of Cardiovascular Disease: A Historical Perspective'. *Lancet*, 2004;383:999–1008.

5. Kevin O'Malley remained as co-director of the BPU until 1990, when he resigned to become Registrar of the RCSI. E. O'Brien. 'History of the Blood Pressure Unit at the Charitable Infirmary and Beaumont Hospital 1978–2006'. *Heartwise*, Winter 2006, pp.12–18.
   The scientific publications from the BPU have been deposited in the Medical History and Scientific Archive of The O'Brien/Lam Collection in the James Joyce Library of University College Dublin.

6. K. O'Malley, E. O'Brien. 'Management of Hypertension in the Elderly'. *New Eng J Med*, 1980;302:1397–1401.

7. E. O'Brien, K. O'Malley. 'The ABC of Blood Pressure Measurement: Future Trends'. *BMJ*, 1979;2:1124–6.

8. E. O'Brien, D. Fitzgerald. 'The History of Indirect Blood Pressure Measurement'. In: *Blood Pressure Measurement*, E. O'Brien and K. O'Malley (eds.), *Handbook of Hypertension*, W.H. Birkenhager and J.L. Reid (Elsevier, 1991).

9. R.E. Beamish. 'Harold Nathan Segall (1897–1990) Profiles in Cardiology'. *Clinl Cardiol*, 1993;16:521–2.

10. M. Laher, E. O'Brien. 'In Search of Korotkoff'. *BMJ*, 1982;285:1796–8.

11. E. O'Brien, D. Fitzgerald, K. O'Malley. 'Blood Pressure Measurement: Current Practice and Future Trends'. *BMJ*, 1985;290:729–34.

12. T.G. Pickering, et al. 'How Common Is White Coat Hypertension?' *Journal of the American Medical Association* 1988;259:225–8.

13. E. O'Brien, J. Sheridan, K. O'Malley. 'Dippers and Non-dippers'. *Lancet*, 1988;ii:397.

14. R. Conroy, E. O'Brien, K. O'Malley, N. Atkins. 'Measurement Error in the Hawksley Random Zero Sphygmomanometer: What Damage Has Been Done and What Can We Learn?' *BMJ*, 1993;306:1319–22.

15. Lever published experimentation showing that with careful attention to detail the errors in the device could be reduced. W.C. Brown, S. Kennedy, G.C. Inglis, L.S. Murray, A.F. Lever. 'Mechanisms By Which the Hawksley Random Zero Sphygmomanometer Underestimates Blood Pressure and Produces a Non-random Distribution of RZ Values'. *J Hum Hypertens*, 1997;11:75–93. The device, although still occasionally used, is now obsolete.

16. Examples include Alan Murray, a physicist from Newcastle upon Tyne; Stefan Mieke, the director of the Physikalisch-Technische Bundesanstalt; Rick Turner from Quintiles; Osamu Shirasaki from the Omron Corporation; Gerhard Frick from MicroLife.

17. STRIDE BP is a non-profit organization based in Athens. Under the guidance of a board of international experts, it provides regularly revised lists of accurate devices to the members of hypertension societies across the world. G.S. Stergiou, E. O'Brien, M. Myers, P. Palatini, G. Parati. 'STRIDE BP: An International Initiative for Accurate Blood Pressure Measurement'. *J Hypertens*, 2020;38:395–9.

18. E. O'Brien, D. Bouchier-Hayes, D. Fitzgerald, N. Atkins. 'The Arterial Organ in Cardiovascular Disease: Arterial Disease Assessment, Prevention, and Treatment (ADAPT Clinic)'. *Lancet*, 1998; 352: 1700–2.

19. The BPU received financial support from Servier Laboratories, a French pharmaceutical company that had been founded by Dr Jacques Servier. Laurent Perret, president of research and development at Servier, facilitated the establishment of the Servier Chair in UCD. In recognition for his support to the BPU and to Ireland, the Royal College of Physicians of Ireland awarded Jacques Servier an honorary fellowship in the Irish Embassy in Paris.
Denis McCarthy, who was Chairman of the Charitable Infirmary Charitable Trust and of Beaumont Hospital, supported applications for funding over many years. E. O'Brien. 'Appreciation: Denis McCarthy'. *The Irish Times*, 9 August 2010.

20. The Board of the CIHC included Cyrus Vance, Boutros Boutros-Ghali, Peter Tarnoff, Daniel Boyer, Rev Joseph A. O'Hare, Abdulrahim Abby Farah, David Owen, Jan Eliasson,

Peter Hansen, Francis Mading Deng and Richard Goldstone. I resigned from the Board in 2020.

21. Land mine essays written by E. O'Brien included: 'The Land Mine Crisis: A Growing Epidemic of Mutilation'. *Lancet*, 1994;334:1522; 'Clearing the Fields: Solutions to the Global Land Mines Crisis'. *BMJ*, 1995;310:1213; 'Clearing the Killing Fields'. *J Roy Coll Phys London*, 1995;25:357–60; 'The Land-Mine Disaster: An Epidemic of Mutilation'. *J Irish Coll Phys & Surg*, 1996;25:54–60; 'Walk in Peace: Banish Landmines from Our Globe'. *BMJ*, 1997;315:1456–8; 'Land Mines' in S. Lock, J. Last, G. Dunea (eds), *Oxford Illustrated Companion to Medicine* (Oxford University Press. 2001), pp. 462–4.

22. 'The Diplomatic Implications of Emerging Diseases'. Symposium on Preventive Diplomacy. United Nations. New York, 23–25 April 1996. Organized by the Center for International Health and Cooperation (CIHC). Chairman: Secretary General Kofi Annan. Proceedings were published in K.M. Cahill (ed.), *Preventive Diplomacy: Stopping Wars Before They Start* (Basic Books, 1996). See also: E. O'Brien: 'Can History Save Us?' *Dublin Review of Books*, 1 July 2021.

23. K. Sabbagh. 'Michael O'Donnell Obituary.' *The Guardian*, 26 April 2019.

24. S. Lock. 'The Achievement of Michael O'Donnell'. *BMJ*, 1982;274:370.

25. Richard McLelland Leech qualified at Trinity College, Dublin, and began working semi-professionally as an actor at The Gate, Dublin, under its directors Mícheál Mac Liammóir and Hilton Edwards, for whom he made his debut as a Nubian slave in *The Vineyard*. He starred in numerous films but always retained his love for medicine.

26. Examples of publications were: 'Six Years Shalt Thou Labour.' *World Medicine*, March 1979; 26–7; and 'Where Have All the Clinicians Gone?' *World Medicine*, 8 March 1978, pp. 30–31.

27. Petrie and I collaborated in hypertension projects among which was a video on blood pressure measurement for the British Hypertension Society. I followed his advice to hand over routine duties in cardiology and to concentrate on developing new methodologies for managing cardiovascular disease.

28. E. O'Brien. 'East Mediterranean Medical Congress'. *Ir Med J*, 1972;65:234.

29. E. O'Brien. 'What Is a Professor?' *Ir Med J*, 1979;72:358.

30. E. O'Brien. 'In Dublin's Fair City. Walter Somerville: The Early Days'. *Br Heart J*, 1981;45: 5–8.

31. E. O'Brien. 'Towards Being a Scientific Doctor and the Dangers of the Dublin Disease'. *J Ir Coll Phys & Surg*, 1982;12:71–4.

32. E. O'Brien. 'The Royal College of Physicians on Kildare Street'. *J Ir Coll Phys & Surg*, 1989;18:128–39.

33. E. O'Brien. 'Strike and the Medical Profession'. *Ir Med J*, 1987;80:247–8.

34. For articles on closure of the journal, see: *Ir Med J*, 1987;80:335–6; *BMJ*, 1988;296:733–4; *JAMA*, 1989;261:1543–5; *Lancet*, 1987;330:1442.

35. E. O'Brien. 'The Island of Dilmun'. *J Ir Coll Phys & Surg*, 1989;18:6–7.

36. The 2011 delegation comprised two doctors, Damian McCormack and me; three politicians, Averil Power, Senator of the Irish Parliament, David Andrews, former Minister for Foreign Affairs, and Marian Harkin, MEP; two members of Front Line Defenders, Andrew Anderson and Khalid Ibrahim; and a photojournalist, Conor McCabe.

37. E. O'Brien. 'Hippocratic Oath'. *Irish Examiner*, 2 August 2011, p.13; E. O'Brien. 'Bahrain: Continuing Imprisonment of Doctors'. *Lancet*, 2011;378:1203–4; E. O'Brien. 'The Weight of Concern' in: *The Weight of Compassion*, pp. 234–6.

38. The term 'corruption of privilege' is used in an article by C. Friedersdorf in *The Atlantic* in 2019 but I had credited the term to Paddy McEntee in 2012: E. O'Brien, *The Weight of Compassion and Other Essays* (The Lilliput Press, 2012), p. 179.

39. See Appendix II: Published Books.

40. See Appendix I: Archives.

41. E. O'Brien, *Conscience and Conflict: A Biography of Sir Dominic Corrigan, 1802–1880* (The Glendale Press, 1983).

42. E. O'Brien, A. Crookshank, G. Wolstenholme, *A Portrait of Irish Medicine: An Illustrated History of Medicine in Ireland* (Ward River Press & RCSI, 1984).

43. The video is in the O'Brien/Lam Collection in UCD.

6. LITERARY DUBLIN

1. Many of the references and quotations in this chapter are from a personal diary covering the years 1976 and 1977, and from papers and correspondence in my possession.

2. The magnitude and diversity of the Baggotonian movement can be appreciated from a listing of the dominant figures in literature, theatre, the visual arts, and music. E. O'Brien, 'The Baggotonian Movement: Nevill Johnson (1911–1999)'. In: G. Dawe, D. Jones, N. Pelizzari (eds), *Beautiful Strangers: Ireland and the World of the 1950s* (Peter Lang AG, 2013), pp. 87–111.

3. I have depended on the following books by Brendan Lynch, from which I have quoted frequently with his kind permission: *Parsons Bookshop: At the Heart of Bohemian Dublin, 1949–1989* (The Liffey Press, 2006); *Prodigals and Geniuses: The Writers and Artists of Dublin's Baggotonia* (The Liffey Press, 2011); *City of Writers: The Lives and Homes of Dublin Authors* (The Liffey Press, 2013); *There Might Be a Drop of Rain Yet: A Memoir* (Mountjoy Publishing, 2022).

4. J. Banville, *Time Pieces: A Dublin Memoir* (Hachette Books Ireland, 2016), p. 3

5. T. Kilroy. 'The Irish Writer: Self and Society, 1950–80'. In P. Connolly (ed.), *Literature and the Changing Ireland* (Colin Smythe, 1982), p. 186.

6. P. Kavanagh. 'If Ever You Go to Dublin Town'. In: A Quinn (ed.), *Collected Poems* (Penguin Classics, 2005), p. 191.

7. B. Lynch, *Parsons Bookshop: At the Heart of Bohemian Dublin, 1949–1989* (The Liffey Press, 2006), p. 195.

8. When I visited the area in March 2022, I was shocked by how Waterways Ireland has allowed this patch of literary history to be despoiled by dilapidation and the daubing of graffiti on the walls and even on the lock gates. The natural clay of the towpath and other areas is smothered with that ever-convenient tool of modernity: tarmac. Most tragically, the original bench erected in 1968 has not been maintained. This little oasis of literary history should be restored to the former beauty that inspired writers and brought serenity to a multitude of troubled souls.

9. J. Ryan, *Remembering How We Stood* (The Lilliput Press, 1987, pp. 123–6) lists the committee.

10. David Davison provided me with his personal recollection of Kavanagh: 'Sadly my final encounter with Kavanagh was on the day after his death at the end of the following November, when I went to the nursing home in Herbert Street where he was laid out in a large room and photographed him from as many angles as possible in the hope that the pictures would be an aid for any future sculptural project. Many years later, when working on the illustrations for *The Beckett Country* and capturing the canal-side view of the nursing home where Beckett's mother died, it occurred to me that she breathed her last in the very same room as Kavanagh.' See also: Obituary: 'Elinor Wiltshire – photographer, botanist and artist'. *The Irish Times*, 6 May 2017.

11. E. O'Toole, B. Lynch (eds), *A Poet in the House: Patrick Kavanagh at Priory Grove* (The Lilliput Press, 2021).

12. A. Cronin, *Dead as Doornails* (The Lilliput Press, 1999), p. 79.

13. B. Lynch, *Parsons Bookshop: At the Heart of Bohemian Dublin, 1949–1989* (The Liffey Press, 2006), p. 29.

14. E. O'Brien. 'A Memory of Micheál Mac Liammóir (1899–1978).' *BMJ*, 1978;3:181–7.

15. E. O'Brien, *Nevill Johnson: Artist, Writer, Photographer* (The Lilliput Press, 2014). In this book, *The Other Side of Six*, revised by the author, is republished. When first published in 1984, it failed to achieve recognition because the publisher, Academy Press, went into liquidation and, despite good reviews, the book disappeared from circulation.

16. The painter was Thurloe Connolly. See: Obituary: 'Thurloe Conolly – A talented artist who liked to paint "things invisible to see"'. *The Irish Times*, 30 April 2016.

17. Anne Yeats, who was probably in love with Johnson, assisted him in producing his photographic record of Dublin city.

18. N. Johnson, *Dublin: The People's City. The Photographs of Nevill Johnson, 1952–53* (Academy Press, 1981). This selection of photographs was published in 1981 (thirty years after they had been taken) with a preface by Nevill and a foreword by James Plunkett. This publication was flawed by poor reproduction of the photographs. Nevill sold the photographic collection to RTÉ, which holds the copyright on the archive. Twenty selected photographs have been reproduced to a high standard with the original preface in: E. O'Brien. *Nevill Johnson 1911–1999. Artist, Writer, Photographer* (The Lilliput Press, 2014).

19. D. Hall in *Nevill Johnson: The Dublin Legacy*. (Ed. E. O'Brien.) Anniversary Press. Dublin. 2014. p. 12.

20. E. O'Brien. *The Beckett Country: Samuel Beckett's Ireland* (Black Cat Press and Faber & Faber, 1986). p. xix.

21. N. Johnson, *Exhibition of Paintings and Drawings*, Solomon Gallery, Dublin, 22 May to 7 June 1995. Opened by E. O'Brien. Programme introduction by S.B. Kennedy.

22. Eugene was renowned for the talent of ventriloquy. He entertained generations of children with puppet shows in a theatre on Clifton Lane at the rear of his house. His TV show *Wanderly Wagon* was an innocent precursor to the intrusion of social media on childhood lives. He was an enthusiast for artistic endeavour, especially in the visual arts.

23. Sheridan was born in County Meath in 1912. He studied literature at UCD and worked with the Irish Tourist Board and RTÉ. He has left a legacy of erudite and revealing interviews with authors of the time, including a remarkable discourse with Sylvia Beach in 1962. He wrote

short stories and scripts for radio and television and with Donagh MacDonagh wrote *Twenty Poems*. A play, *Seven Men and a Dog*, was produced by the Abbey Theatre in 1958.

24. Monica Sheridan became a celebrity cook with a TV programme entitled *Home for Tea*. Her methods were irregular, not least her frequent licking of her fingers as she concocted a badly rehearsed dish. She won a Jacob's Award in 1965 for 'putting personality into cooking' and published two cookbooks, *Monica's Kitchen* and *The Art of Irish Cookery*.

25. Malcolm Arnold began his musical career as a jazz trumpeter but soon devoted himself to composition, writing nine symphonies and many concertos. He wrote music for contemporary musicians including Julian Bream, Julian Lloyd Webber, Benny Goodman and Larry Adler. He wrote the scores for many films, including *The Bridge on the River Kwai* and *The Belles of St Trinian's*.

26. N. Jeffares, 'On a Fallen Electrician', *The Poems & Plays of Oliver St John Gogarty* (Colin Smythe Ltd, 2001), p. 353.

27. The limerick in question was: 'There was a young man from St John's / Who wanted to roger the swans / Oh no! said the porter, / Please oblige with my daughter, / The birds are reserved for the dons.' The poetic conundrum for the Nobel laureate and the hallowed company was simply whether the last line should read 'For the swans are reserved for the dons.' As happens when events are passed on from memory rather than from written documentation, details of the recalled event may differ and the correct description of the event may never be known. Sheridan's depiction of the discussion on the limerick states that Yeats indulged in conversation with George Russell (AE), whereas J.B. Lyons records that the discussion was between Yeats and George Moore; there are also differences between Lyons and Sheridan on the actual wording of the limerick. We can merely surmise from the perspective of hindsight, and allowing for the language of the time, that Yeats indulged in conversation with either Moore or Russell on the most appropriate wording of the last line of a limerick written by Gogarty. See: J. B. Lyons. Oliver St. John Gogarty. Dublin Historical Record. 1984;38:2–13. N. Jeffares, 'The Young Man from St. John's', *The Poems & Plays of Oliver St John Gogarty* (Colin Smythe Ltd, 2001), p. 352.'

28. N. Sheridan. Doctors and literature. *BMJ*, 1978;ii:1779-1780

29. D. Johnston. Waiting with Beckett. *Irish Writing*. 1951;23-28

30. Salvador Dalí claimed: 'I'm a very bad painter. Because I'm too intelligent to be a good painter. To be a good painter you've got to be a bit stupid.'

31. O'Doherty had sipped sherry and listened intently to the advice of the older man, whom he sketched six weeks before his death in 1957. He later donated this sketch to the Yeats Museum in the National Gallery of Ireland. Samuel Beckett also visited Yeats in the Portobello Nursing Home, though he and O'Doherty never met. The minimalism that both men sought to bring to their work was probably influenced by Yeats. See Brenda Moore-McCann, *Brian O'Doherty/Patrick Ireland: Between Categories* (Lund Humphries, 2009).

32. The tourist publicity for the house reads: 'For an astonishing change of pace, visit the Painted House. The house can be visited by appointment contacting Elisa. Flat entry fee of €30 for up to 6 people; additional guests €3 each.'

33. Brian created no less than four alter egos – Sigmund Bode, Mary Josephson, William Maginn and most famously he adopted the pseudonym Patrick Ireland in protest from distant New York to the shooting of unarmed citizens in Derry on Bloody Sunday.

34.   B. O'Doherty and J. Stanley in *Hello, Sam*. Christina Kennedy (ed.). Irish Museum of Modern Art. Published retrospectively to document the exhibition *Hello, Sam* (2011) as part of Dublin Contemporary, 17 September–29 October 2011.

35.   The interview video, which was recorded on 21 June 2011, was lost for years but is now in the Brian O'Doherty Archive of the O'Brien/Lam Collection in the Special Collections Department of the James Joyce Library in UCD.

36.   Obituary notices in *The Irish Times*, *New York Times*, and many other newspapers on 23 Nov 2022. Also: E. O'Brien. 'Appreciation', *The Irish Times*, 28 November 2022.

37.   Petr Skrabanek was born on 27 October 1940 in Náchod, Czechoslovakia. He studied chemistry, entering Charles University in Prague in 1957. In 1963 he studied medicine at Purkyně University and in 1967 was selected to spend a month in Galway Regional Hospital where he met his future wife, Vera, in July 1968. This was the year of the Soviet invasion of his country and Skrabanek suddenly found himself homeless. With help from several people sympathetic to his predicament, most especially Harry O'Flanagan, the then Registrar of the RCSI, he was admitted to the College to finish his medical studies. He qualified in 1970 and for the next four years worked in neurology in various Dublin hospitals. In 1975 he joined the Endocrine Oncology Research team in the Mater Hospital as a Senior Research Fellow and became involved in research into the neurotransmitter agent known as substance P.

38.   P. Skrabanek, J. McCormick, *Follies and Fallacies* (Tarragon Press, 1989). P. Skrabanek, *The Death of Humane Medicine and the Rise of Coercive Healthism* (Social Affairs Unit, 1994).

39.   Richard Walsh was a scholar, linguist, and phoneticist, who had had a brilliant academic career at UCD. Gerald Victory produced 200 works, including four symphonies, eight operas, a large-scale cantata, two piano concertos and a large volume of other compositions, many of them written for films, plays and celebratory occasions.

40.   I visited Long in his impoverished studio in Werburg Street and was glad to be able to help him financially in the very straitened circumstances in which he lived. Long died from cancer in 2016 at the young age of fifty-two years.

41.   The Skrabanek translation can be assessed in the Maldoror archive in the O'Brien/Lam Collection in UCD. The archive also contains documentation relating to the Dublin translation of *The Cantos of Maldoror* together with studies for illustrations and a catalogue of John Long exhibitions and details of the Skrabanek Foundation.

42.   O'Mahony. 'Petr Skrabanek: The Abominable No-man'. *J Royal Coll Phys Edinburgh*, 2019;49:65–9.

43.   I have consulted the following works:
       Books of poetry: *The Lundys Letter*; *Sunday School*; *Points West*; *Micky Finn's Air*; *Ethna MacCarthy: Poems* and *The Last Peacock*. Books of criticism and comment: *In Another World: Van Morrison & Belfast*; *The Wrong Country: Essays on Modern Irish Writing*; *The Sound of the Shuttle: Essays on Cultural Belonging & Protestantism in Northern Ireland*; *Catching the Light*; *Views & Interviews*; and *Beautiful Strangers: Ireland and the World of the* 1950s. A Memoir: *Looking through You.*

44.   E. O'Brien, 'The Baggotonian Movement: Nevill Johnson (1911–1999)'. In G. Dawe, D. Jones, N. Pelizzari (eds), *Beautiful Strangers: Ireland and the World of the* 1950s (Peter Lang AG, 2013), pp. 87–111.

45. E. O'Brien. *The Weight of Compassion & Other Essays* (The Lilliput Press, 2012),

46. E. O'Brien, G. Dawe (eds), *Ethna MacCarthy: Poems* (The Lilliput Press, 2019).

47. R. Ballagh, *Robert Ballagh: A Reluctant Memoir* (Head of Zeus, 2017).

48. Patrick Kavanagh. 'I Had a Future in Antoinette Quinn (ed.), *Collected Poems* (Allen Lane, 2004), p. 186.

49. Ibid. 'News Item', p. 239.

50. E. Morgan. '€15m for Gothic Manor on 19 Acres'. *The Irish Times*, 29 September 2005.

51. I was cardiologist to the Rotunda Hospital, which was close to the Jervis Street Hospital, an arrangement that enabled me to be there in minutes and have patients transferred for cardiological care if required.

52. Ben wrote delightful notes after our meetings: "Eoin, mo Chara, Did I ever get to thank you for the gift of the great Beckett book. If not let me do so now, like a whore in Bundoran. Every good wish to Tona and yourself. After 75 it is all uphill Or downhill?' This is a reference to Beckett's acknowledgment of the rejection of *Murphy* by the American publisher Doubleday, Doran: 'Oh Doubleday Doran / More oxy than moron / you've a mind like whore on / the way to Bundoran.'

7. PARISIAN INTERLUDE

1. See, for example: E. O'Brien, *The Beckett Country: Samuel Beckett's Ireland* (Black Cat Press and Faber & Faber, 1986); E. O'Brien (ed). 'The Writings of A.J. Leventhal' in *A.J. Leventhal 1896–1979: Dublin Scholar, Wit and Man of Letters*, Leventhal Scholarship Committee (The Glendale Press, 1984); Samuel Beckett, *Dream of Fair to Middling Women*, E. O'Brien and E. Fournier (eds) (Faber & Faber, 2020).

2. Ethna MacCarthy is the protagonist in many of Beckett's writings, most notably the early poems such as 'Alba', fiction including 'A Wet Night' and *Dream of Fair to Middling Women* and the play *Krapp's Last Tape*. E. O'Brien, G. Dawe (eds), *Ethna MacCarthy: Poems* (The Lilliput Press, 2019), p. vii.

3. Quotations attributed to Niall Montgomery are from: 'Abraham Jacob Leventhal: A Eulogy.' In: E. O'Brien (ed), *A.J. Leventhal 1896–1979* (Con Leventhal Scholarship Committee and The Glendale Press, 1984).

4. Bonham's catalogue. 'Lot 205. Beckett (Samuel). Beckett collection of Marion Leigh, partner of Beckett's intimate friend A.J. ('Con') Leventhal.' London, 20 June 2018.

5. E. O'Brien, 'From the Waters of Sion to Liffeyside: The Jewish Contribution: Medical and Cultural.' *J Ir Coll Phys and Surg*, 1981;10:107–19.

6. *The Klaxon*, Winter 1923–4 and *To-morrow*, Vol. 1, No. 1, August 1924; Vol 1, No. 2, September 1924.

7. The Leventhal Scholarship Committee: B. Wright, J. Weingreen, S. Beckett, N. Sheridan, N. Montgomery, A. Woolfson, M. Leigh, T. Murtagh, C. Simon, F. Barry, H. Jay, J. Jay, G. Davis, B. Moss, K. Adams, D. Hayter, A. Madden, M. Senior, B. Coyle, H. Jameson, P. McEntee, M. Fehsenfeld.

8. *Thirty Years of the A.J. Leventhal Awards: 1984–2014*. Long Room Hub, Trinity College Dublin, 22 January 2015.

9. See Appendix I: Archives.

10. Le Tiers Temps is the retirement home at 24–26 rue Rémy Dumoncel in Paris, where Beckett spent his last years. The name is the title of a novel by Maylis Besserie translated into English by Clíona Ní Ríordáin and published by The Lilliput Press in 2022 with the title *Yell, Sam, if You Still Can.*

11. E. O'Brien, 'Samuel Beckett et le poids de la compassion'. *Critique*, Août–Septembre 1990;519–20; 641–53. This would become the title of a collection of essays published by The Lilliput Press in 2012, *The Weight of Compassion & Other Essays.*

12. S. Beckett, *Dream of Fair to Middling Women*, E. O'Brien, E. Fournier (eds) (Black Cat Press, 1992, Faber & Faber, 2020).

13. Examples are: *James Joyce et la création d'Ulysse* by Frank Budgen and *La Mort que l'on se donne* by Aidan Higgins.

14. Fournier's translations include: *Bande et Sarabande* [*More Pricks than Kicks*] (Les Éditions de Minuit, 1995); *Trois Dialogues* (Les Éditions de Minuit, 1998); *Quad et autres pièces pour la television, suivi de l'Épuisé par Gilles Deleuze* (Les Éditions de Minuit, 1999); *Les Os d'Echo et autres précipités* (Les Éditions de Minuit, 2002); *Cap au pire* [*Worstward Ho*] (Les Éditions de Minuit, 2012); *Peste soit de l'horoscope et autres poèmes* (Les Éditions de Minuit, 2012); *Proust* (Les Éditions de Minuit, 2013).

15. I am grateful to Natalie Pigeard Micault for these details and a copy of the obituary notice for Georges Fournier Senior, which acknowledges both the humanitarian ethos that motivated him and his skill as a doctor.

16. The death notice in *Le Monde* read: '*Stella Fournier Ailaud, sa soeur et sa famille, Son frère, Son beau-frère, Ses neveux et nièces, Irène Lindon, la famille Murphy, ses amis et ses soignants, tous ceux qui l'ont connue, ont la tristesse de faire part du décès de* EDITH FOURNIER, *amie et traductrice de Samuel Beckett, survenu le Dimanche 24 avril 2022, à l'âge de quatre-vingt-sept ans. L'inhumation a eu lieu au cimetière du Montparnasse, Paris 14. Cet avis tient lieu de faire-part et de remerciements.*'

17. Ernst Hans Josef Gombrich (1909–2001), Austrian-born British art historian.

18. Beckett's forty-six cards and notes to me from August 1976 to September 1989 have been donated to the Beckett Archive in The O'Brien/Lam Collection in the James Joyce Library in UCD.

19. G. Craig, M. Dow Fehsenfeld, D. Gunn, L. More Overbeck (eds), *The Letters of Samuel Beckett 1966 to 1989* (Cambridge University Press, 2016).

20. HAPPY DAYS Enniskillen International Beckett Festival, 22–26 August 2013, with contributions from Tariq Ali, Tom Paulin, Margaret Drabble, Anthony Cronin, John Montague and Eoin O'Brien.

21. J. Knowlson, 'Foreword' in E. O'Brien, *The Beckett Country: Samuel Beckett's Ireland* (Black Cat Press and Faber & Faber, 1986), p. xvii.

22. S. Beckett, 'Hommage à Jack Yeats' in *Disjecta: Miscellaneous Writings and a Dramatic Fragment* (John Calder, 1983), p.149.

23. S. Beckett. *Krapp's Last Tape* in *Samuel Beckett: The Complete Dramatic Works* (Faber & Faber, 1986), p. 219.

24. The Tyrone Guthrie Centre. This retreat was managed with efficiency by Bernard and Mary Loughlin. Mobile phones had not been invented and telephonic communication was possible only by dialling Newbliss 2, where the telephonist joined silently (apart from her wheeze) in every conversation. Writing was only disturbed by the gentle plop of cowpats in the field below my window. Colm Tóibín was also in residence, and we shared many evenings discussing Beckett.

25. The special-edition signed pages, which were brought to Paris by James Knowlson and signed by Beckett, read; 'This edition of *The Beckett Country* is limited to 250 numbered and 10 lettered copies all of which have been signed by Samuel Beckett. The binding for the edition was devised by Tona O'Brien and executed by Des Breen of Antiquarian Bookcrafts. Specially printed with spot-varnishing of the photographs on Jupiter 143 gsm matt satin-finish paper by Arnoldo Mondadori Editore Italy the edition is hand-bound in full grey goatskin on which the larch-tree emblem of Beckett's childhood from a drawing by Robert Ballagh is embossed in gold. The furze-yellow authentic water-silk end-papers and the slip-case on which the larch-tree emblem is embossed blind depict the yellow bells of mountain gorse.'

26. *The Beckett Country* received good reviews across the world with a consensus being that Beckett scholarship would now have to take account of the inspirational effect of place and past, that the Irish influence in Beckett's oeuvre would have to be recognized

27. *Dream of Fair to Middling Women*, Samuel Beckett's first novel, was written at the Hôtel Trianon in Paris, during the summer of 1932 when the author was twenty-six years old. It had remained unpublished until the Black Cat Press published it sixty years later in 1992.

28. These documents are lodged in my archives in TCD. See Appendix I: Archives.

29. B. O'Doherty and J. Stanley. *Hello, Sam.* Christina Kennedy (ed.). IMMA. Published retrospectively to document the exhibition of *Hello, Sam* (2011) as part of Dublin Contemporary, 17 September–29 October 2011.

30. Anonymous. Francis Evers. Obituary. *The Irish Times.* 18 September 1996.

31. My personal correspondence with Barbara Bray has been placed in my archives in TCD. See Appendix I: Archives.

32. Herman Braun-Vega, 1984. *Catalogue Paysages – Mémoires.* Maison Internationale du Théâtre Renaud-Barrault. Théâtre du Rond-Pont, Paris, 1984.

33. Anne Atik, *How It Was: A Memoir of Samuel Beckett* (Faber & Faber, 2001). Alba Arikha, *Major/Minor* (Quartet Books, 2011).

34. G. Dukes. 'Beckett Memoirs Not Made of This'. Review of 'How It Was: A Memoir of Samuel Beckett' by Anne Atik. *The Independent*, 24 November 2012.

35. D. Johnson. Obituary. Jérôme Linden. *The Guardian*, 17 April 2001.

Appendix I: Archives

Papers, correspondence, notes and memorabilia relating to various parts of the text have been donated to the following archives. Many of these items have been archived and are available for research; the process of formal archiving is in progress for remaining items.

JAMES JOYCE LIBRARY AT UNIVERSITY COLLEGE DUBLIN

The O'Brien Lam Collection in the Special Collections of the James Joyce Library at UCD consists of the following archives:

- *The Beckett Collection*: Correspondence, papers, photographs and memorabilia relating to Samuel Beckett, *The Beckett Country* publication and the *Photographic Exhibition of The Beckett Country*.
- *The Nevill Johnson Archive*: Correspondence, writings, paintings and memorabilia relating to the artist, photographer and writer Nevill Johnson.
- *The Medical History & Scientific Archive*: Correspondence, writings, and a large photographic collection relating to the history of Irish medicine.
- *The Smiddy Archive*: Correspondence, papers, photographs and memorabilia relating to Timothy Aloysius Smiddy, Envoy Extraordinary and Minister Plenipotentiary of the Irish Free State to the United States. This archive also contains papers and documents donated by Eda Sagarra, who wrote the biography of her grandfather, *Envoy Extraordinary: Professor Smiddy of Cork* (Dublin: Institute of Public Administration, 2018).

THE LIBRARY OF TRINITY COLLEGE DUBLIN

The following archives have been established in the Library of Trinity College Dublin:

- *The Eoin O'Brien AJ Leventhal/Ethna MacCarthy Collection*: Correspondence, papers, photographs and memorabilia relating to A.J. Leventhal and Ethna MacCarthy.
- *The Eoin O'Brien Samuel Beckett Collection.* Correspondence, papers, photographs and memorabilia relating to Samuel Beckett and Parisian associates.

UNIVERSITY OF LIMERICK

The following items have been donated to the University of Limerick Art Collections:

- The Art History Library of Eoin O'Brien
- Nevill Johnson (1911–99), *GOLGOTHA*, 1995. Acrylic on board.

ROYAL COLLEGE OF PHYSICIANS OF IRELAND (RCPI)

Eoin O'Brien Research Papers ACC/1983/2. Papers and correspondence of Eoin O'Brien relating to his research and publications on Sir Dominic Corrigan. Catalogued by Harriet Wheelock, June 2011.
See: https://rcpi-live-cdn.s3.amazonaws.com/wp-content/uploads/2018/01/Eoin-OBrien-Research-Papers.pdf

ROYAL COLLEGE OF SURGEONS IN IRELAND (RCSI)

Donations of papers, books, and miscellaneous instruments are presently being assembled for archiving in the Historical Collections of RCSI.
See: https://www.rcsi.com/dublin/library/collections

SENATE HOUSE LIBRARY, UNIVERSITY OF LONDON

Photocopies and papers, c. 1992, relating to the publishing difficulties involving Samuel Beckett's *Dream of Fair to Middling Women* (Black Cat, Dublin, 1992), Edith Fournier and Eoin O'Brien (eds). [Reference code(s): GB 0096 MS 931]

LEXICON LIBRARY, DÚN LAOGHAIRE-RATHDOWN COUNTY COUNCIL PUBLIC LIBRARIES, HAIGH TERRACE, MORAN PARK, DÚN LAOGHAIRE, CO. DUBLIN

Collection of original and copied photographs of coastal photography in both physical and digital formats, books and papers relating to the coastal area of South County Dublin.

MUSEUM OF LITERATURE IRELAND (MOLI), NEWMAN HOUSE, ST. STEPHEN'S GREEN, DUBLIN.

Selection of mounted photographs from *The Beckett Country* and posters of the international displays of *The Beckett Country Exhibition*.

EMBASSY OF IRELAND, 2234 MASSACHUSETTS AVE NW, WASHINGTON, DC 20008, USA

Limoges tea set, which was in the possession of Muriel O'Brien, is now on display in the Irish Embassy in Washington with the inscription: 'This Limoges tea set belonged to Professor Timothy Smiddy, Ireland's first diplomatic envoy to Washington (1924–29). It was presented to the Government of Ireland by his grandson Eoin O'Brien.'

THE ARTHUR HOLLMAN COLLECTION, BRITISH CARDIOVASCULAR SOCIETY, 9 FITZROY SQUARE, LONDON W1T 5HW

Two ECG machines, mercury sphygmomanometers and stethoscope.

Appendix II: Published Books

The following books on personalities and institutions have been written and/or edited by E. O'Brien:

Essays in Honour of J.D.H. Widdess. Edited by E. O'Brien. City View Press. Dublin. 1978.

Conscience and Conflict: A Biography of Sir Dominic Corrigan 1802–1880. The Glendale Press. Dublin. 1983.

A.J. Leventhal 1896–1979: Dublin Scholar, Wit and Man of Letters. Edited by E. O'Brien. Leventhal Scholarship Committee. The Glendale Press. Dublin. 1984. This book lists the items for auction and contains an essay by Niall Montgomery entitled 'Abraham Jacob Leventhal: A Eulogy', an essay by Abraham Jacob Leventhal entitled 'Samuel Beckett: A Note', and a bibliographical compilation entitled 'The Writings of A.J. Leventhal: A Bibliography', which lists forty-six articles and criticism written by Leventhal between 1922 and 1978, together with a complete listing of fifty-eight contributions he made on a regular basis to the *Dublin Magazine* from 1943 to 1958.

The Royal College of Surgeons in Ireland 1784–1984. The Irish Heritage series. Eason & Son. Dublin. 1984.

A Portrait of Irish Medicine: An Illustrated History of Medicine in Ireland. E. O'Brien, A. Crookshank, G. Wolstenholme. Ward River Press & RCSI. Dublin. 1984. Also Limited Edition.

The Charitable Infirmary, Jervis Street 1718–1987: A Farewell Tribute. Edited by E. O'Brien. Anniversary Press. Dublin. 1987.

The House of Industry Hospitals 1772–1987: The Richmond, Whitworth and Hardwicke (St. Laurence's Hospital). A Closing Memoir. Edited by E. O'Brien, L. Browne, K. O'Malley. Anniversary Press. Dublin. 1988.

The Bicentenary of The Royal College of Surgeons in Ireland, 1784–1984: Proceedings. Edited by K. O'Malley, E. O'Brien. The Glendale Press. Dublin. Two Volumes. 1987.

Messiah: An Oratorio by George Frideric Handel. Programme notes compiled and edited by E. O'Brien. The Black Cat Press. Dublin. 1986.

The Beckett Country: Samuel Beckett's Ireland. The Black Cat Press, Dublin. Faber & Faber. London & Boston. 1986. Also special edition signed by Samuel Beckett.

The Beckett Country: Catalogue of an Exhibition for Samuel Beckett's Eightieth Birthday. E. O'Brien, J. Knowlson. The Black Cat Press. Dublin. 1986.

The Royal College of Physicians of Ireland. Anniversary Press. Dublin. 1989.

Nevill Johnson, 1911–1999: Paint the Smell of Grass. D. Hall, E. O'Brien. Ava Gallery 2008.

Nevill Johnson: The Dublin Legacy. Anniversary Press. Dublin. 2014.

Nevill Johnson: Artist, Writer, Photographer. The Lilliput Press. Dublin. 2014.

Ethna MacCarthy: Poems. Edited by E. O'Brien, G. Dawe. The Lilliput Press. Dublin. 2019.

Seapoint: Sea, Sky and Spires. Anniversary Press. Dublin. 2017.

A Century of Service: The City of Dublin Skin and Cancer Hospital, 1911–2011. Anniversary Press. Dublin. 2011.

The Weight of Compassion & Other Essays. The Lilliput Press. Dublin. 2013.

Index